THE BEST OF JAIL MEDICINE

AN INTRODUCTION TO THE PRACTICE OF CORRECTIONAL MEDICINE.

Jeffrey E. Keller, MD

Dedication

To Angela. She has been the motor and brains of our correctional medicine career from the beginning. Without her there is no JailMedicine.

Acknowledgements

I would like to acknowledge the following individuals who provided advice, inspiration, and guidance. *The Best of Jail Medicine: An Introduction to Correctional Medicine* would not have been possible without their help. Thank you, thank you to the following!

Lorry Schoenly, who led the way with her excellent blog Correctionalnurse.net and her many books and timely advice.

The American College of Correctional Physicians, especially Christine and Brian Westbrook, for their enthusiastic sponsorship.

Mike Puerini, who first had the idea of writing such a book and transferred that idea to me.

Todd Wilcox, who has taken over responsibility for the Jail Medicine blog since my retirement.

The many people at Badger Medical who supported and contributed to the Jail Medicine blog, especially Brian Mecham, Kim Ammons, and Shyra Been.

My mentors and friends who provided inspiration and support, especially Jane Haddad, Sharen Barboza, Paul Wilde, Gary Raney, Steve Shelton, Tom Groblewski, and Al Cichon.

Thank you to John Erich for editing, Chris Cebollero for help with publication, and, most especially, my business partner and wife, Angela Keller.

ADVANCE PRAISE

The Best of Jail Medicine: An Introduction to Correctional Medicine is an incredibly valuable distillation of years of knowledge practicing in this unique niche of medicine. It is on-point for many of the difficult decisions that we must make, it is insightful, it is funny, and shortens the learning curve for anyone new to this field. This is a much-needed resource that has been a long time in development. I am so thrilled that this resource exists now for all of the clinicians who currently work and will work in this field. Anyone practicing in this field of medicine will find this book to be an invaluable resource. I recommend it as an important resource for how to work effectively in a correctional healthcare setting.

Todd R. Wilcox, MD, MBA, FACCP, CCHP-A, CCHP-P
Medical Director, Salt Lake County Jail System

For years, little guidance existed about the practical aspects of delivering care within a correctional setting; we all had to learn it along the way with bumps and lumps that trial-and-error entails. In 2012, Dr. Keller took the initiative to create the *JailMedicine* blog to fill that gap. He knew instinctively what we were all longing for – a clear, concise, no-nonsense approach to understanding how to navigate healthcare delivery in jails and prisons. *The Best of Jail Medicine: An Introduction to Correctional Medicine* is filled with nuggets of wisdom that will save healthcare professionals working in corrections not only time, but the mental gymnastics of untangling what you cannot see. From withdrawal, operations, and medical care to the corrections-specific issues of comfort items and patient behavior, Dr. Keller provides new and seasoned clinicians alike with helpful and usable insights.

Sharen Barboza, Ph.D. Clinical Psychologist

TABLE OF CONTENTS

I. Introduction

How Did I End Up in Jail?.. 2

II. Overview

Correctional Medicine Is a Great Job 6

Incarcerated People Can't Shop 10

Jails vs. Prisons... 13

My Jail Is Safer Than Your ER.................................. 18

Who Pays Inmates' Medical Bills? 21

III. Care and Communication

Meeting New Patients in a Jail 26

The Principle of Fairness 29

All Clinical Encounters Are Discussed Back in the Dorm........... 33

Our Patients Can't Be Fired...................................... 36

Our Patients Don't Go Home 40

Don't Be the Decider... 45

Words Matter.. 47

IV. Operations

I Came to See the Doctor... 52

Medical Clearance... 55

Outside Physicians 57

Medical Necessity... 61

The Compliance Trap.. 63

Utilization Management Is Different in Corrections 66

Patient Satisfaction... 69

Grievance Responses 74

How to Write an Alternative Treatment Plan.................... 79

V. Comfort Items: The Special Problem of Correctional Medicine

Comfort Items 86

Personal Shoes.. 89

Don't Do Doubles 92

Eyeglasses and Eye Exams.. 96

VI. Withdrawal

Thoughts on Alcohol Withdrawal 102

Opioid Withdrawal Can Be Deadly 106

Opioid Withdrawal... 109

Benzodiazepine Withdrawal..................................... 113

The Most Common Mistake When Treating Withdrawal........... 116

VII. Medical Care

Beware the Bounce-Back.. 120

Medical Refusal or Manipulation 123

Documenting Test Results.. 130

Patient Weight Is a Powerful Diagnostic Tool 133

An Approach to Chronic Pain 136

Food Allergies 139

VIII. Behavior

Manipulation 146

Handling the Manipulation of Confrontation............ 148

Is My Patient Faking? 151

The M-Word—Malingering 153

Chemical Sedation vs. Physical Restraint................... 160

IX. Opinions

The Meaning of Medically Necessary 166

COVID-19 Fatigue and Leadership 170

A Concrete Cell for the Mentally Ill......................... 172

How Lawsuits Drive Correctional Medicine.............. 175

Can the Raiders Be Saved Using the Principles of Medical Research?. 178

About Author.. 182

INTRODUCTION

How Did I End Up in Jail?

So let's get the big question out of the way first: How on earth did I, a respectable physician, wind up practicing medicine in a freaking jail, of all places? Well, the answer is that it was a fortunate accident.

Nobody aspires in medical school to practice in a prison or jail. Neither did I. Like most physicians who practice in jails and prisons (collectively termed *correctional medicine*), I ended up here quite by accident.

I am an emergency physician by training. I had been happily working at a busy emergency department for about 10 years when my local county commissioners approached me to ask if I would be willing to take over medical services at the small local jail. My initial response was, "What are you, nuts? Who'd want to work in a jail?" Many of you probably would have said the same thing! Fortunately for me the commissioners gave me a second chance six months later. I was still leery, but I told them I'd do it for one year and one year only.

Two things happened during that year, though. First I discovered I liked working at the jail (and who would have thought that?!). In many ways it was like working in an ER. In fact, many of the "frequent flyers" from the ER also were regular attendees at the jail. I'd often see people in the jail clinic I'd seen days earlier in the ER. Or I'd see someone in the ER and ask, "So when did you get out of jail?"

In addition, though, I saw a lot of needy people in the jail who did not routinely come to the ER. For many people jail is the first time they've had easy access to medical care. I saw medical issues that had been neglected for years. A typical exchange would be, "What do you think of this growth on my hand?" "Well, that's cancer." I'm not sure what I had naively expected, but what I found was a lot of untreated interesting medical pathology. I've

The Best of Jail Medicine

diagnosed bacterial endocarditis several times (lots of IV heroin users go to jail). I've diagnosed syphilis. Within a couple of months, I had treated more people for alcohol withdrawal than I had in my entire ER career. I felt good about what I was doing. Weird!

Second, my phone kept ringing. "We're the jail just up the road. We need help too!" "We're the jail down the road. We need a doc." It turns out there are a lot of jails, but there aren't a lot of physicians raising their hands to volunteer for jail medical duty. I was practically the only guy in my home state of Idaho who was. After a few years I'd accumulated so many small jails that I retired from the ER to do jail medicine full time. And Idaho is not the only place with a need for correctional medicine practitioners.

There are presently around 2.1 million incarcerated people in the United States, and they all need healthcare. In fact, incarcerated people are the only residents of the U.S. with a constitutional guarantee of it. The Supreme Court ruled in 1976 that to deny necessary medical care to incarcerated people constituted cruel and unusual punishment. Because of this ruling every correctional facility, even a tiny county jail with only 10 beds, must have some program in place to provide medical, dental, and mental healthcare to its incarcerated population. No wonder my jails were so eager to find a willing medical practitioner!

One other thing happened, though, when I began to practice jail medicine full time: I became almost invisible to the rest of the medical community. When I was in the ER, I bumped shoulders with the other medical staff all the time. Now, though, the only time I see my colleagues is when I run into them at the grocery store. And when I tell them I left the ER to work in jails full time, I often get quizzically raised eyebrows. I can see them thinking, *What are you, nuts? Who'd want to work in a jail?* Their next question, though, is typically, "What is it like?"

The thing is, I like working in jails. I was never unhappy as an ER physician. But I get more overall satisfaction out of my work in jails and prisons.

OVERVIEW

CORRECTIONAL MEDICINE IS A GREAT JOB

Before I knew anything about correctional medicine, I had a bad opinion about it. I'm not proud of this. I even turned down my first opportunity to get into correctional medicine because of this prejudice. Thank goodness I got a second opportunity, because correctional medicine changed my life! Who knew it could be such a great job and career?

Certainly not my colleagues. Back when I made the midlife career change, my bewildered physician friends asked me, "Why in the world would you want to work in a jail?" Without knowing anything about it, they had a preconceived notion of correctional medicine being low-skill and basically without redeeming features.

What a difference 15 years makes!

I recently ran into an acquaintance, an anesthesiologist, at a community function. "How are things going in the jail?" he asked.

"Great!" I said. "I was never unhappy as an ER physician, but I have much more job satisfaction now than I did then. I have a great job!"

"You're lucky," he said. "I hate my job." He went on to discuss hassles with billing, reimbursements, fights with hospital administrators, boredom, and other problems.

This was not an unusual occurrence. I've had similar conversations with several physician friends. I know an orthopedic surgeon who hates his job and wants to retire—but can't afford to. Another acquaintance is an internist. "Insurance and billing are killing me!" he told me. "I'm forced to see many more patients an hour than I'd like. I can't give my patients the time or attention they deserve." Another internist and a family practitioner I know gave up their longstanding practices to become hospitalists—but they don't love that job, either. The list goes on and on.

I think I can safely say a large percentage of physicians in the outside medical world are unhappy in their work. This is borne out by satisfaction surveys. Typically a third of practicing physicians would not choose a career in medicine if they were offered a do-over. Half would not recommend medicine as a career to their children! Only a third rate their morale as good or excellent.

Yet a switch to correctional medicine is not on any of these physicians' radar! Just like I did, outside physicians tend to have a distrust of correctional medicine. They don't know anything about it, but they don't like it. But that is the key: *They don't know anything about correctional medicine!*

And that's too bad because, as I found out, correctional medicine is a great career. We just need to get the word out.

Benefits

As I was thinking about what makes correctional medicine a great career, I came up with the following:

Correctional medicine frees you from coding, billing, and insurance companies.

Outside physicians can spend more than 15% of their gross revenues just on coding, billing, and collections. Then there are the hassles and headaches of dealing with recalcitrant insurance companies. One of my friends calls this "The tyranny of the Blues" (meaning Blue Cross and Blue Shield, with whom he's had plenty of frustrations). Total overhead for a primary care practice can be as high as 70% of gross revenues.[1]

My own experience practicing in an emergency medicine partnership was similar. Over 20 years billing became more complicated (have you seen the size of ICD-10?), insurers became more aggressive, and revenues fell.

But correctional medicine is different. Correctional medicine is a fee-for-access model, rather than the fee-for-service model used in the outside world. This means there is no ICD-10 coding. We don't bill insurance companies. We don't do "wallet biopsies," and we don't send patients to collections. We're free, free, free! I found this to be a huge benefit when I made the transition. I would never want to go back to the coding and billing world.

You'll get to see much more medical pathology in corrections than you do now.

In jails we see lots of acute pathology. One example is that jail physicians are the true experts in assessing and treating acute withdrawal syndromes, like those with alcohol and heroin. I bet I personally have treated more patients for acute withdrawal than all the noncorrectional physicians in Idaho put together.

Jails also see many people who are disenfranchised from outside medicine. These are the patients who have no insurance, no money—maybe they're homeless—and many never go to a doctor no matter how sick they get. The jail medical clinic may be the first medical care to which they've had easy access. And, of course, they bring an impressive array of untreated maladies. I've newly diagnosed everything from cancer to diabetes to rheumatoid arthritis in patients with no doctor on the outside.

Prisons present another unique opportunity: In outside medical practice it is rare to be able to follow a patient's progression over many years. Medicine has become so specialized that patients pass from doctor to doctor, depending on what disease they develop.

Take, for example, the case of a primary care doc in a local community who has been taking care of a particular patient, Joe, for 20 years. Then say Joe develops lung cancer and renal failure. There is a good chance Joe will now be cared for by an oncologist and nephrologist. His primary care doctor may never see him again!

However, in a prison, Joe (and patients like him) will always return to his primary correctional physician after each visit to a specialist. As a result we get to watch the course of his disease progression and response to therapy in a way not done in the outside world. Couple that with the fact that every type of weird pathology you can imagine is found in our prison population, and we can confidently say we in corrections get to see much more interesting medical pathology than most other physicians.

For the most part, correctional medicine is 9–5, weekends and holidays off.

This was a big deal for me, an ex-emergency physician. For the first time in 25 years, I rediscovered regular circadian sleep. Who knew that would be so great? Also, I was no longer gone every other Christmas and Thanksgiving. Lovely!

Remember those doctors who gave up their primary care practices to become hospitalists? They gave up their practices due to coding, billing, and insurance hassles. But now, as hospitalists, they sacrifice their sleep and holidays. That is one reason they still aren't happy. Plus they miss having long-term relationships with patients. If only there were a career path that had it all.

There is: correctional medicine! They just have never been told. It is up to us to get the word out.

Reference

1. Catanese SJ; Western PA Healthcare News Team. Understanding the Complexities of Overhead in a Physician Practice. Western Pennsylvania Healthcare News. Published August 7, 2013

INCARCERATED PEOPLE CAN'T SHOP

Incarcerated people cannot go out to find good doctors in their communities. Good doctors have to choose to go to them!

I remember the first time someone told me I was "wasting my talents" by working in a jail. At that time I had no ready witty rebuttal. I love my job, and I especially appreciate working with a patient population that is disadvantaged and underserved. Of course, even the idea that incarcerated people are worthy of medical care may be *controversial.* Incarcerated people are not as politically correct as other medically disadvantaged populations.

As an example, if you were to tell your family and friends you were going to work at a clinic for the homeless in an inner city or provide care in a needy third-world country, their reaction probably would be along the lines of, "Good for you! I admire your selflessness and dedication!" Yet when you tell these same people you're going to work in a prison, you are much more likely to get, "Why would you waste your talents working with them?"

I have heard the "wasting your talents" line more than once, and it is a double insult. It assumes that people who are incarcerated do not deserve medical care. It also assumes that if you are going to work in a jail or prison, there is something wrong with you.

I've tried to think about why otherwise good and kind people often have this reaction to the notion of providing medical care to those in jails and prisons. Upon reflection I believe it is an emotional response based on the following assumptions:

1. People are incarcerated as a punishment.
2. So they don't deserve good medical care.

3. Therefore, jail and prison medical providers, like you, must be there specifically to *not* provide good medical care. What kind of doctor does that?

4. Also, everyone I see portrayed on TV and in the movies who works in prisons is a loutish brute. Maybe you are a loutish brute too.

5. I'm basically fearful of the whole idea of jails and prisons. I don't want to think about it.

In the end if you go to work in a jail or prison, your reputation may suffer. Colleagues may look at you askance. You may become stigmatized.

But it should not be that way! All these assumptions are incorrect.

Let's look at the incarcerated population more objectively, using terms that could be assigned to other medically disadvantaged groups considered worthy.

Disadvantaged—Of course incarcerated people are disadvantaged. That's what going to prison is all about—losing normal societal privileges. However, one right people in jails and prisons do not lose is the right to necessary medical care.

Underserved—Yes, incarcerated people, as a group, are underserved. Doctors are not lining up to work in prisons! It is not atypical for correctional medical positions to go unfilled for long periods. In fact, that is how I initially got involved in corrections. My county commissioners couldn't find any medical doctor to staff the local jail for months! Thank goodness they finally asked me.

Disenfranchised—People incarcerated in jails and prisons are beyond disenfranchised. They have been formally banished from society. In fact, one reason for negative reactions to the announcement "I'm going to work in a prison" is that by doing so we break the unwritten social rule that *we've agreed not to associate with those people. Those people,* of course, are those incarcerated in jails and prisons. That's what people mean when they say, "You're wasting your talents."

People think this about incarcerated people and mean it. But if, instead of incarcerated inmates, *those people* you are referring to are some other large social group—like women or immigrants or Muslims—the statement is instantly recognizable as blind prejudice. The incarcerated seem to be the only social group against whom prejudice and contempt are socially acceptable.

In the end incarcerated people are indeed socially disadvantaged. They cannot go out to find good doctors in their communities. Good doctors have to choose to go to them. Incarcerated people have that in common with many people in the third world, where a medical mission may be the only medical care available.

So, if you want to do work that is socially meaningful, working with patients who are socially marginalized and lack ordinary access to medical care, you could volunteer to work at a third-world clinic. You could work in a similar medical clinic in an inner city. Or you could instead go to work in a jail or prison! I have to say, this kind of medicine can be pretty gratifying.

We correctional professionals need to embrace the fact that we work with a disadvantaged and marginalized population. When a fellow physician says, "You work in a jail?" with one eyebrow raised, we need to say back, "Of course I work in a jail! That's where the sick and needy people are! Why aren't you working in a jail?"

The Best of Jail Medicine

JAILS VS. PRISONS

I was talking to a physician colleague one day who was quite interested in what I was doing and in correctional medicine in general. Like most people he had no idea what the difference was between jails and prisons and what the practice of medicine was like in the two settings. While the term *correctional medicine* encompasses both jails and prisons, the actual practice of medicine in the two settings can be as different as an emergency department and a nursing home.

A good way to illustrate the difference is by using patients as models. To this end consider two patients entering the correctional system for the first time, a homeless alcoholic and a successful middle-aged businessman who sees his primary care physician regularly.

The first important difference between jails and prisons is that jails tend to get patients "fresh off the streets."

Take the case of Randy. Randy is a homeless alcoholic who was drunk and aggressively demanding money from people downtown. Now he's charged with disturbing the peace. As you might expect, Randy has not seen a doctor in a long time, both because he has no health insurance and because, besides his alcoholism, he has an underlying mental illness that makes him paranoid. When Randy receives his medical intake screening at the jail, he is found to have lice and a weeping open wound on his foot. His blood sugar is 450. After eight hours in the jail, Randy also begins to show signs of alcohol withdrawal.

Patients like Randy are not uncommon in jails. Jails see and treat many patients going through all sorts of withdrawal syndromes, from alcohol to narcotics like heroin to cocaine and bath salts. Even if they have no substance abuse issues, many jail patients haven't been receiving regular medical care before coming to jail. Perhaps they are one of the 30%–40% who have no health insurance. Or maybe they just haven't been taking care of themselves. It's not uncommon to see patients show up in the jail medical clinic with uncontrolled diabetes or untreated hypertension. Since this is perhaps the first time they've had easy access to medical care, jail patients will often ask providers to look at other chronic problems they've worried about for years. Finally, like Randy, many jail patients have serious untreated mental illnesses, and many are in jail because they have acutely decompensated.

Since Randy was arrested on a relatively minor offense, he will eventually be released from jail. Although jails typically do what they can to help patients like Randy with social problems like homelessness, many end up back in the same situation until their next arrest. Jails commonly see many such "revolving door" patients who go through withdrawal each time they return to jail and only get medical care for their other chronic conditions while there.

Were Randy to be charged with a felony, the situation would change significantly, since he would likely not be released from jail before he's eventually sent to prison. This highlights the difference between jails and prisons.

While prisons can see similar off-the-street problems such as withdrawal, neglect, and untreated mental illness, these are much less common in prisons than jails. The reason is that most patients with these problems will have spent a significant amount of time in jail awaiting trial and sentencing before they are sent to prison. Were Randy to eventually end up in prison, his alcohol withdrawal should be long past, his lice eradicated, his wound healed, and he should have begun treatment for his diabetes and mental illness.

The second important difference between jails and prisons is that people tend to go to jail for much shorter lengths of time than those who go to prison.

Jails basically house two types of people. The first are those who have been charged with crimes but not yet had their guilt or innocence determined by the courts. These are the "innocent until proven guilty." They are in jail not as a punishment but to guarantee they will show up in court. Depending on when their court appearance is scheduled, these people may only be in jail overnight, or they may sit in jail awaiting trial for months if they cannot pay the bail amount set for their release.

Second, jails house people sentenced by the courts to serve time for misdemeanors. In general these sentences can be no longer than one year and usually are much shorter, sometimes as short as a couple of days. Because of this the average length of stay in a typical jail usually is only 2–3 weeks, with a few getting out almost immediately and others staying for many months.

Prisons, on the other hand, only house people who have been found guilty of felonies and subsequently sentenced to prison. In general, the shortest amount of time any person will be sentenced to serve in prison is one year, and usually longer. Some will remain in prison for the rest of their lives.

These factors make a big difference in the medical approach to patients. Take, for example, the case of John. John is a successful 50-year-old businessman charged with embezzlement. He has a physician he sees regularly and who prescribes him medications.

Since John will be able to pay the bail set by the court, he probably will only be in jail for a short amount of time, days or weeks, and then return to his outside doctor. Many jail patients are like John, and in most cases like this, jail medical providers will not make major changes to John's medical treatment. Even if John is prescribed, say, an iffy blood pressure medication most practitioners wouldn't normally use, they probably would not change it. It will just get changed back when John is released!

Instead, a main goal of jail medicine is maintaining continuity of medical care from the community to the jail and back. We don't want John to have a disruption of his prescribed medications when he comes to jail or when he leaves. This can sometimes be tricky, especially if John didn't bring his medications to jail with him and can't remember exactly what he's supposed to take.

Since there are so many patients like John entering and leaving in a short amount of time, having a system to ensure continuity of medications is a big deal in jails. Sometimes, as well, new jail patients like John may have doctor visits or procedures scheduled for while they are incarcerated. Jail practitioners often have to sort out what is important for patients to go to despite being in jail (like dialysis) and what can be rescheduled until they get out (like routine wellness visits).

This situation would change were John to be sentenced to prison. In this case he will not be returning to his outside doctor anytime soon, if ever. The prison medical staff will be taking over his medical care lock, stock, and barrel. This situation is like a person moving to a new city and needing to find a new medical provider there. Like this new practitioner, the prison medical staff is under no obligation to continue any medical treatments they think are unwarranted or ineffective. In fact, like a new provider in a new city, they may want to start from the beginning by reevaluating what John's current medical problems are, prescribing medications (which may or may not be the same as what he was on before), and setting up a long-term treatment plan that includes scheduled chronic care clinic visits for hypertension and diabetes and routine wellness procedures like colon cancer screenings. Since there are many patients like John in the prison system, these routine chronic care follow-up visits and wellness checks are common, much more so than in jails, and all prisons must have a system for scheduling and monitoring them.

It turns out that after a few years in prison, John is found to have metastatic colon cancer and needs both chemotherapy and radiation treatment. This is not an uncommon scenario in prisons. Since many people are sentenced to very long terms, prisons accumulate many patients who develop severe chronic illnesses, such as cancer, kidney failure, paralysis, Alzheimer's dementia, and every other condition you can think of. Prisons must do a lot of "end of life" planning jails almost never have to deal with. Managing chronic disease conditions from the mundane (like hypertension) to the serious (like coordinating a bone marrow transplant) is common in prisons but not jails.

Of course, these are generalizations. There is a lot of overlap between what jails and prisons do. Jails sometimes have patients who remain there for years, just not as many as prisons. And prisons may have newly arrived patients who go through alcohol or opioid withdrawal, just not as many as jails.

Of course, most other aspects of correctional medicine are almost identical whether you're in a jail or a prison: Clanging doors, security, and "sick call" clinics are prime examples.

After hearing my explanation about medicine in jails and prisons, my friend wanted to take a tour of the local jail. I think this is a great idea. Our colleagues need to have a better idea of what we do! They need to know what happens when their patients go to jail or prison.

My Jail Is Safer Than Your ER

People naturally assume working in jails and prisons is dangerous. "Aren't you nervous about working there?" they ask me. What people have seen of jails on TV looks pretty rough! After all, that's where they put the violent criminals, right? The problem is, it just isn't so!

Jails and prisons are not dangerous places to work; to assume so is just one of many misconceptions people have about correctional facilities. In fact, my jail medical clinics have been a much safer work environment than where I worked before.

I worked in a busy ER for upward of 25 years. During that time I was slapped, punched, and kicked—several times—and had to wrestle with many out-of-control patients.

I was spat upon. A patient peed on my leg. I was pooped on (don't ask). One patient pulled a knife on a colleague in a small exam room. My colleagues and I found a good number of guns while cutting clothes off trauma victims. And guns were found hidden in the waiting room!

Though I witnessed no shootings during my ER years (thank goodness), gunfire in emergency departments across the country has not been uncommon, and staff members have been among their victims.

But interestingly, no one ever said to me during my ER days, "Wow! Aren't you nervous about working in that dangerous ER?" That is because most people have been in an ER and so know from experience that overall, they aren't really dangerous places. On the other hand, most people have never been in a correctional facility. All they know about jails and prisons is gleaned from movies and books. And in movieland, danger sells.

So how dangerous are my jail medical clinics? Well, during the 15 years I've worked in correctional medicine, nothing has happened like my

ER experiences—not once! The worst that has happened is that patients have occasionally yelled at me. Some have even called me obscene names.

That all you got? Yawn!

There are several reasons why my jail medical clinics are safer overall than a typical ER:

1. Weapons are forbidden in correctional facilities. The jail deputies don't carry guns while on duty. This isn't because they don't carry firearms; just like patrol officers, detention deputies are issued service weapons and expected to carry them when not in the jail, even when not on duty. But when detention deputies come to work, they secure their weapons in lockers at the jail entrance. No guns are allowed in the facility at all! Most jails and prisons require all employees and visitors to go through airport-like metal detectors to make sure no weapons end up in the jail.

2. People in jails and prisons are, for the most part, sober when I see them. It is hard to stress how important this is! The worst patients in the ER were those who were drunk, belligerent, and wanting to fight. Patients in the jail clinic have sobered up and are less belligerent.

3. Even if a jail patient wants to fight, I don't have to be involved. Burly detention deputies are always nearby. Though we try to safeguard patient privacy as much as possible, in jails safety and security take precedence. This means security staff are always close, so they can respond immediately. During most clinical encounters in my jails, the detention deputy is situated just outside the room to allow some privacy but still be able to respond immediately if something happens. If a patient has a high enough risk level, one deputy (or even two) may stand right next to me.

4. Incarcerated patients are punished for acting out in clinics. This rarely happens in ERs. But in jails the punishment is no joke. Ill-behaving patients can lose privileges (like not being able to buy from the jail commissary or the loss of visitation rights), be transferred to maximum-security status, or even face additional criminal charges. Nothing dissuades bad behavior more than swift and sure consequences!

5. Lastly, I can terminate clinic appointments knowing I can see the incarcerated patient again in a day or even in a couple of hours. He

is just in his cell down the hall. This is my go-to response to someone swearing at me: "We're done now, but I'll see you again in a little while after you've calmed down." In the ER I had to put up with bad language, because if I kicked a patient out of the ER, I might never see them again. That was likely my one and only chance to make the diagnosis.

Of course, I'm not saying violence never occurs in jails, because it does. Far and away, however, most of this involves the security officers, not the medical staff. Thank goodness for them!

Who Pays the Medical Bills for Incarcerated Patients?

One of the more frequent questions I get from people curious about jail medicine is, "Who pays for this? And how do you get paid?" Well, correctional medicine certainly has a different payment and reimbursement system than we use for the rest of American medicine. In fact, those incarcerated in jails and prisons have a medical system that has more in common with Canada's single-payer model than the U.S.

The central fact upon which correctional medical care hinges is this: Incarcerated people are the only residents of the United States with a constitutional guarantee of medical care. I say *residents* rather than *citizens* because the guarantee of healthcare while imprisoned applies to illegal immigrants as well as U.S. citizens. There is no such guarantee for the rest of us who reside freely in the U.S. If we free citizens want medical care, we have to figure out some method of paying for it. Most of us do this by obtaining some type of insurance, usually through our employer or the government.

However, it is rare for an incarcerated person to have private insurance. Also, people lose the right to use any federal insurance plan when they're incarcerated. By law, Medicaid and Medicare benefits (with few exceptions) cannot be used while incarcerated. Incarcerated people also lose veteran benefits and even active-duty military insurance. We can't take a jailed veteran, for example, to his next VA clinic appointment. He is no longer eligible to use the VA system, even to get his medications refilled.

Instead, every correctional facility must set up its own independent medical program paid for by whatever entity is in charge of the jail. Counties pay directly for the medical care of people incarcerated in their jails. Each state pays for the medical care of its state prisoners. And the federal government funds care for patients in federal prisons. Any way you look at it, these are your tax dollars at work!

The federal prisons and about half the state prison systems hire the nurses, counselors, dentists, doctors, etc. they need to staff their services as federal or state employees. The other half of states have privatized their prison medical services and so negotiate with correctional health companies to provide them. Jails have a similar breakdown, although the bigger the jail, the more likely it is to be privatized.

This unique (for the U.S.) system of providing medical care in jails and prisons makes correctional medicine different in many important ways from care in the free world.

What this system means for the incarcerated is that they all have equal access to medical services. There are no "haves" and "have-nots" like there are in the outside world. Incarcerated patients don't have to do anything to be eligible for benefits other than be incarcerated. In this way correctional medicine resembles socialized medicine, like in Canada.

The only time my patients reenter the world of fee-for-service medicine is when they need specialty care that cannot be provided in the jail or prison medical clinic. As an example, say a jail patient breaks his hand in a fight and needs surgery. The orthopedist would submit her bill to the county for payment like she would bill the insurer of any other patient.

What this direct payment system means for me is that I am paid a flat fee for my jail services, a fee I negotiated with the sheriff and county commissioners. Doctors in state prisons are paid a set salary for what typically is a 9–5 job. There are no fee-for-service charges for any of us. We don't bill Medicaid or Blue Cross for doing a physical exam or any procedures. From my perspective, I love it! I'm freed from the tyranny of DRGs (diagnosis-related groups) and those damn ICD-10 codes I hated in my previous medical life. I can't overstate how wonderful this is for my personal satisfaction with my career.

Another important difference between this system and outside medicine is that there's a budgeted ceiling for medical expenditures. For example, consider a typical state prison system. The legislature budgets a certain amount of money for the Department of Corrections, including the prison facilities, the salaries of correctional officers, and the money to run medical services. Included therein is the money to pay for patients on dialysis, as well as money for cancer chemotherapy and the drugs for hepatitis C. It is all included. There can be a lot of pressure on correctional physicians to count pennies. I don't think this is necessarily a bad thing.

Physicians on the outside generally don't have to worry about counting pennies or any budget ceiling. An outside physician can prescribe the new, expensive biologics advertised on TV to one patient without having any impact on her other patients. This is not true in a prison system. If prison docs use a super expensive medication with an iffy benefit profile for one patient, that means there's less money for mundane but important stuff like treating type 2 diabetics. Correctional medical administrators wrestle with these types of trade-offs all the time, as well as routinely having to lobby state legislators for more money for the medical needs of incarcerated patients—not a top legislative priority, I can tell you!

The United States has two very different medical systems—one for free citizens and the other for incarcerated residents. Compared with the rest of the world, the way we fund medical care for incarcerated patients is less weird than the rest of the U.S. medical system.

CARE AND COMMUNICATION

Meeting New Patients in a Jail

I'll be meeting a new jail patient with multiple medical problems today in my clinic. I know this much before I meet him: He will almost certainly be scared, especially if this is the first time he's been to jail. He will likely be suspicious of me. He may even be downright hostile. I know this because this is the norm for correctional medicine. I can't be an effective doctor unless I can turn this attitude around.

Consider the situation from my patient's perspective. Prior to seeing me he was arrested, handcuffed, and driven to jail in a police car. Once at the jail he was thoroughly searched (spread-eagle against the wall), fingerprinted, and had his mug shot taken. His clothes were taken away, and he was given old jail clothes (including used underwear). He was placed in a concrete cell. Now he's summoned by a correctional deputy and told (not asked) to go to the medical clinic.

He did not choose me to be his doctor. Though he doesn't know anything about me, he has no choice but to see me for his medical care. Not only did he not choose me, but he also cannot fire me or see anyone else. He may fear I am not a competent doctor—otherwise, why would I be practicing in a jail?

This is the attitude I have to overcome. How to do this is an essential skill for correctional practitioners. And of course the single most important encounter is the first one. A negative first impression is hard to overcome— and I'm already starting at a disadvantage. What I must do in only a few minutes is convince my patient I'm a legitimate medical doctor and care about him. I have learned in many years of doing this that these things are essential:

I must put aside my judgments, emotions, and fears. I will be taking care of people accused of horrific crimes, such as pedophilia, murder, and rape. But I am now their doctor and must do my best to take care of their medical needs. If I feel disgust, I must not show it or allow it to interfere with my judgment. Similarly, I will find other jail patients frightening, and still others I will genuinely like. I cannot allow these emotions to show in my affect or behavior, either. A basic principle of correctional medicine is fairness. I must treat all patients the same, whether I like them, fear them, or am repelled by them.

I must look like a doctor. If I want this patient to trust my competence and judgment, I need to look the part. There is a temptation to think, *Hey, it's a jail! I don't need to dress up!* But that is a mistake. If I dress casually in jeans, a t-shirt, and sandals, it will confirm my patient's unconscious suspicion that I am not a "real" doctor. When I worked in the ER, I usually wore scrubs, but since jail patients commonly wear scrublike attire, scrubs are out (in my opinion). I personally usually wear a dress shirt, slacks, and a suit coat. Appearance for a healthcare provider is more important in a jail, not less.

I must be genuine and gentle. It may be that my patient has not heard a kind word since being arrested. Being in jail can be humiliating. New patients will assume I am also going to be stern. I should treat the introduction as if I were meeting this person in church, not a jail. If I look the patient in the eye, smile (genuinely), and say "Hi, Mr. Smith! I'm Dr. Keller. It's nice to meet you," or "It's good to see you again," this will go a long way toward establishing a working doctor-patient relationship instead of an inmate-jail employee relationship.

I should get close, if possible. If I start out behind my desk (where I was reviewing the patient's chart before they arrived), I need to come out so there is no barrier between us. Yes, security is important, but I should not act as if I am afraid of my own patient. Besides, since there is always a security officer nearby, the actual risk of violence is less than that of the average emergency department.

I need to explain my role. I usually say my job is to continue their medical care while they are in jail. A common fear of new jail patients is that I am going to take over and ignore what their previous doctor has done. I tell my new patients I'm going to work with their outside doctors. Sometimes this only entails reviewing old medical records. However, a phone call to their outside practitioner will go a long way in establishing trust with my new patient. I may indeed eventually take over if the patient stays in jail long enough, but hopefully I will have established a good and trusting doctor-patient relationship by then.

I need to explain how medical care in jails works. There are not a lot of advantages to being in jail generally, but one exception—a true advantage in most jails—is how accessible medical care is. Patients with chronic medical problems are generally seen by medical personnel more frequently in jail than they would be on the outside. For example, if they take medications, they will come face-to-face with a nurse every day. It is easy to frequently check blood pressure, blood sugars, and weight and schedule "how are you doing?" sorts of visits. I tell my new patients, "I'll be talking to you a lot!"

I need to be patient. Even with a good start healthy relationships are not (of course) made in a single visit. It typically takes several weeks, many visits, and patience to get patients to consider me to be *their* doctor. But it does happen!

THE PRINCIPLE OF FAIRNESS

I'm often asked by my noncorrectional colleagues what it's like to work in a jail. I tell them practicing correctional medicine is different in many ways than medicine in the "free" world. Many of them scoff at this. How could the practice of medicine be different in a jail than anywhere else? "Medicine is medicine," they say.

But correctional medicine is different. In my experience, if you just throw a practitioner into a jail or prison clinic without any training, he likely will not do well. It took me two full years before I was comfortable in my sick-call clinics, and I learned new things constantly. Experience matters in corrections!

This is obvious to those of us who have experience working in jails and prisons. But how do you explain the intricacies of a jail medical clinic to an outside physician? I've thought about this a lot over the many years I've practiced correctional medicine, and I've come up with several concrete examples of how correctional medicine is different from medicine "on the outs." The first and perhaps most important difference is the principle of fairness.

The Principle of Fairness

In my opinion, the first and most important difference between correctional medicine and outside medicine is that in corrections we must be fair and uniform in our treatment of jail patients. We need to treat all our jail patients the same. This is very different than the way medicine is practiced outside of jails. Outside medicine is not fair at all. Examples are easy to point out.

The first is that what kind of medicine you get in the outside world depends on how wealthy you are and what quality of medical insurance you have. Walk into (almost) any doctor's office or clinic in the U.S., and the first procedure performed will be the "wallet biopsy." If you have no insurance or inferior insurance and no money, you likely will be turned away. With no insurance you often can't afford to buy your prescribed medications.

I ran into this dilemma repeatedly when I was an emergency physician. I would discharge an uninsured patient with instructions to follow up with a physician in the community, only to learn later that the physician had refused to see them without cash up front. Variations of that happened more times than I could count. Often there was no one in my community who would see an indigent ER patient.

This dilemma continues to happen in jail clinics! I once had a patient arrive with type 1 diabetes. We got it under control while he was incarcerated, but upon his release, despite numerous phone calls, no local practitioner was willing to continue to take care of him without payment in advance—which the patient did not have.

I understand this. Outside medical practice is a business, and like any business, if a medical practice were to treat patients for free, it wouldn't remain in business for long. Also, there are federal rules that say if a practitioner offers discounts to one patient, they must also offer that discount to Medicare and Medicaid patients. So even if physicians are willing to treat some patients pro bono, it is illegal to do so.

I've been talking here about uninsured patients, but even patients with lesser-quality insurance are discriminated against by some practitioners. I know of physicians who refuse to accept Medicare and Medicaid. You could be a patient of a certain doctor I know for 30 years, but the second you turn 65, you will receive a letter discharging you from their practice. True!

Also, some practitioners refuse to accept negotiated price schedules from insurance companies and so are not "preferred providers." This, of course, means their patients may not see those physicians without up-front cash payments.

In the end outside medicine is, well, not fair! The "haves" can get any care they need or want, while the "have nots" must accept limited choices or nothing at all.

That is, unless they go to jail or prison!

As we in the correctional medicine business know, people who are incarcerated have a constitutional guarantee to medical care. They are the only U.S. residents I am aware of who have this guarantee. Note that I used the word *residents* rather than *citizens,* because the right to medical care applies to everyone who is incarcerated, whether a citizen of the United States or an illegal immigrant.

The right of the incarcerated to necessary medical care was established in the landmark 1976 Supreme Court decision Estelle v. Gamble. In this decision the Supreme Court held "deliberate indifference to serious medical needs of prisoners constitutes the 'unnecessary and wanton infliction of pain'…proscribed by the Eighth Amendment."

Memorize this line!

Further legal decisions have expanded upon what is meant by this phrase, but in the end all jails and prisons must provide necessary medical, mental health, and dental care to their inmates.

We don't get to do "wallet biopsies." Everybody in our correctional institutions can request to be seen by a practitioner. Everyone is assessed and treated for medical problems, both big, like cancer, and small, like athlete's foot. Both acute, like a sprained ankle, and chronic, like hypertension.

In fact, a big part of our job, especially in prisons, is to make sure patients with problems like hypertension or diabetes don't fall through the cracks and get forgotten. We call that *chronic care.* On the outside, if a patient doesn't show up for his scheduled yearly checkup, the doctor's office might send him a reminder card, but other than that, too bad.

But in a well-run prison, such a patient would not be forgotten. If necessary, medical staff will send a correctional officer to his housing dorm to bring him in for his appointment. He can refuse, but it usually has to be in person and in writing.

Medical Needs vs. Medical Wants

A final issue of fairness between outside medicine and correctional medicine is this: On the outside there is little distinction made between medical needs and medical wants. In fact, some of the most lucrative medical practices are devoted to wants, like aesthetic surgery. Most of the direct-to-consumer advertising of drugs we see on television is (in my opinion) an attempt to make people want drugs they don't need.

In jails and prisons patients have a right to treatment of their medical needs but not their medical wants. A big part of what correctional practitioners do is sort out needs versus wants. One obvious example that will resonate with all correctional providers is the inevitable request by patients for a double mattress. This is a classic want but certainly not a medical need. In fact, this is not a medical issue at all, in my opinion.

The principle of fairness is important in any consideration of a medical want. You cannot give any medical service to one patient and deny that service to others. That creates "special" patients who get special privileges. If you give one patient a medical service, you are obligated to give every patient with a similar presentation the same service.

If a correctional practitioner approves a double mattress for a patient who, say, complains of chronic low back pain, they are bound to approve a double mattress for every patient with a similar complaint.

The consideration of fairness underlies everything we do in correctional medicine. It is hard to overstate how important it is. There is not a day that goes by in my correctional medicine practice where fairness does not come up.

ALL CLINICAL ENCOUNTERS ARE DISCUSSED BACK IN THE DORM

The second big difference between correctional medicine and outside medicine is this: Every clinical encounter in correctional medicine is discussed back in the housing dorm. This does not occur in outside medicine and is critically important to understanding doctor-patient relationships in corrections.

For those not familiar with the housing situation in jails and prisons, most incarcerated people are housed in large housing dorms or pods. Depending on the size of the institution, these can house anywhere from 10 to more than 100 people. As you might expect, people in such dorms spend a lot of time talking with each other, especially since they generally have more free time than your average person in the outside world. Incarcerated people spend *a lot* of time talking to one another.

So when a jail patient returns to the dorm from a visit to the medical clinic, it is natural for the encounter to be discussed. If the encounter was unusual or noteworthy in any way, this quickly becomes known throughout the pod. And since different housing pods also communicate with each other, information about clinical encounters quickly spreads throughout the entire institution.

This does not occur in any meaningful way in the outside world. Back in my emergency medicine days, my ER patients did not call up other ER patients when they got home to discuss their experience. General medicine clinics are the same. The patients in, say, a family practice office do not communicate with each other outside the practice. With few exceptions most don't even know each other.

This strange phenomenon of patients in a medical practice communicating with each other about their experiences is unique to corrections. And it creates a unique dynamic that is critically important to understand to succeed in correctional medicine.

Jail patients know when you're not being fair.

The principle that every clinical encounter is discussed back in the dorm is very closely connected to the principle of fairness.

In outside medicine practitioners routinely favor some patients over others. Here are some examples: Patient A and Patient B call at the same time for an appointment for the same complaint. Patient A is told the next available appointment is in 10 days. Patient B, a personal friend of the practitioner, is told, "Come tomorrow morning, and we'll work you in." In another example, two practitioners work in the same office. Doctor X always gives a splint and Norco prescription to any patient with a sprained ankle. Nurse Practitioner Y, on the other hand, never does. If you have a sprained ankle, how you will be treated depends on which provider you're assigned to. If you present with a sore throat, Doctor X always will give you a prescription for an azithromycin Z-Pak. Nurse Practitioner Y rarely does; she is more likely to talk to you about viruses.

This can work in outside medicine because these patients never talk to each other. But such discrepancies in practice and behavior do not work in correctional medicine because every clinical encounter is discussed back in the dorm! Patient A and Patient B will talk to each other. The ankle sprain patients will compare notes. The patient with a sore throat will wonder *Why didn't I get an antibiotic?*

Correctional practitioners need to keep this principle in mind. Here, for example, is a common scenario from the correctional world. Let's say someone comes to the jail medical clinic and says to a new practitioner, "I have low back pain, and I'm not comfortable on these thin mattresses. I want you to authorize a double mattress." If the practitioner writes the order for the double mattress, this will be discussed back in the dorm. Within days that practitioner is going to see many more medical requests for double mattresses from others, who will say, "I have back pain too! I also want a double mattress." And via the principle of fairness, if you give one patient a double mattress based on a complaint of back pain, you are obligated to give everyone with the same complaint a double mattress if they ask for it. Otherwise, you are treating the first person as special.

Because of their unique situation, incarcerated people can be quite sensitive to issues of perceived unfairness and special treatment. Anytime a medical practitioner does something for one person they don't do for others, the perception of unfairness can manifest with complaints, grievances, and even lawsuits.

Your professional demeanor will be discussed.

Every aspect of a professional encounter is fair game to be discussed back in the dorms. If you dress nicely and like a medical professional, this will be noted and discussed. Other jail patients will come to medical confident they're seeing a true professional. Alternatively, if you do not look the part of a medical professional (stained jeans, sandals, poor hygiene), this also will be noticed and discussed. Your patients will arrive with a poor impression already planted in their minds.

Also, incarcerated people know the security rules of the institution very well. If you violate security rules, this will be discussed back in the pods. If you do a special favor for one person, such as allowing a phone call or giving a gift (example: a piece of candy), others will learn about this and discuss the implications in detail. Other jail patients will invariably ask you to do favors for them as well.

There are no secrets in a jail or prison! Every encounter with medical personnel is discussed back in the dorm. What do you want that discussion to be about?

OUR PATIENTS CAN'T BE FIRED

There's a controversy in pediatrics I've been following recently. Some pediatricians have been dismissing children from their practice if their parents won't allow them to be vaccinated. This practice has been criticized as punishing innocent children for the actions of their parents, but the pediatricians defend it by saying they're just trying to protect their other patients from being exposed to pertussis, measles, and other transmittable diseases in the waiting room.

This story illustrates an extreme example of something we all know: that the practice of "firing" patients is common in outside medicine. Many of my jail patients have been dismissed from medical practices, some more than once. Patients can be fired for variety of offenses. Some violate the contracts of their pain clinics. Some are dismissed for simply not following their doctor's advice—like to get their children vaccinated. Many are no longer welcome when they cannot pay their bills or have lost insurance coverage. Finally, patients can be fired for just being too difficult to deal with. One jail patient I remember screamed drunkenly at his doctor's secretary to the point that she called the police. He received his official dismissal letter while in jail.

Well! Things are different in correctional medicine! We can't fire our patients. Our patients remain our patients no matter what. It doesn't matter if they violate the terms of a pain contract by diverting medications. It doesn't matter if they refuse to follow our advice. It doesn't matter if they're difficult to deal with.

I've had patients in my clinics who became angry and, Hulk-like, swelled up into veritable Roman candles of F-bombs. I don't tolerate this kind of behavior and have deputies escort them back to the housing dorm—

but (and this is a big *but*) *they are still my patients.* I cannot fire them! And I will see them again, hopefully when they're under more control.

Our patients can't fire us either.

The flip side of the same coin is that our patients cannot fire us either. On the outside it's easy to change practitioners. Don't get along with your doctor? She won't give you what you want? There are 10 more just down the street, especially if you have insurance.

We are all familiar with the concept of "doctor shopping," in which a patient (usually drug-seeking) goes to several different practitioners looking for the one that will give him what he wants. Just as common are "doctor accumulators," who go to Doctor A for one complaint, Nurse Practitioner B for a second problem, and so on.

People incarcerated in correctional institutions have lost this ability. The practitioner at that facility is their doctor. They have no say in the matter. Many become frustrated and angry about this situation, especially when the correctional practitioner won't give them what they want. Correctional patients sometimes respond to this by demanding access to different practitioners. This rarely works, though. In the end the practitioner at their facility is the one they have to see, like it or not.

Since jail patients cannot fire their practitioner, they instead will often try to force their practitioner to do what they want using various forms of manipulation. This can range from confrontational verbal intimidation and the threat of lawsuits to flirtatiousness and fawning ("You're the best doctor I've ever known! And the only one who truly understands me!"). Correctional practitioners encounter variations of these behaviors every day. But no matter how egregious such attempts at manipulation may be, we cannot respond by refusing to see the patient. Firing our patients is off the table.

Verbal Jiujitsu

Because we cannot fire our correctional patients no matter how hard to deal with they sometimes are, and because they cannot fire us no matter how frustrated they become, correctional practitioners have to learn techniques for dealing with our difficult patients. I call this *verbal jiujitsu.*

New correctional practitioners *must* know the principles of verbal jiujitsu to do at all well in a correctional clinic. If they do not, clinical encounters will be stressful, unpleasant, and unproductive. There is a high turnover among correctional physicians, and I think one major reason is that many do not have the verbal skills to deflect confrontations. Getting beat up verbally day in and day out eventually becomes intolerable.

It doesn't have to be this way! Like anyone else, jail patients go with what works. For example, if you respond to the threat of a lawsuit by giving in—well, you're going to be threatened with a lot of lawsuits. If you don't have a good strategy for dealing with aggressive verbal confrontation, jail patients will realize that this strategy works with you—and you will see a lot of it in your clinics.

The reward feedback to the patient doesn't even have to involve getting what they want. They can read your body language and demeanor. Just getting you upset may be all the reward they need! In fact, verbal confrontation is simply a habit with many. It is how some people have interacted with just about everybody for their entire lives. In fact, that ingrained confrontational personality disorder is one of the reasons they are in prison in the first place. And just like anyone else who become adept at something by practicing a lot, these people are very practiced and adept at verbal confrontations—much more than you and me.

Verbal jiujitsu is what I call the verbal skills used to deflect and defuse verbal confrontations. Notice I did not say *defeat*. *Defeat* implies a battle, and the whole point of verbal jiujitsu is to *avoid* doing battle.

Take an angry patient like the one described above. There he is, in my clinic, fists clenched, red-faced, and hurling F-bombs. Nurses, deputies, and maybe even other jail patients are watching. What should I do? The usual gut instinct is usually wrong.

Wrong response No. 1, *compromise*: "There's no reason to be angry! Calm down, and we can work something out." Mistake! If you compromise, you've established the precedent that throwing a tantrum and screaming is effective in influencing you to change your mind. Other jail patients will learn this. The result is that you will see others threaten to get angry and wait for you to compromise.

Wrong response No. 2, *angry retaliation*: Don't get right in his face and scream back, "Get out of my clinic! Who do you think you are?!" In this case the jail patient didn't get what he wants, but he did learn yelling at you is an effective way of getting under your skin. Anytime he wants to push your buttons, even if solely for his own amusement, he knows how to do it. Also, you've ruined your own mood for the day. Your heart is jackhammering, you're sweating through your shirt, and you now have a screaming headache (at least that's what would happen with me). There's no good outcome here!

The verbal jiujitsu response is to *defuse* and *deflect*: "We're done for now. Security will take you back to your dorm. We'll talk again later after you've calmed down." It's important to say this without raising your voice and, if possible, to betray no emotion on your face. That way there is no reward for the poor behavior. No compromise, no bargaining, no reaction. In a day or two you can call the patient back to medical and confidently expect better behavior. Plus, since every clinical encounter is discussed back in the dorm, everyone else now knows throwing a fit will not be successful with you. You will see fewer of them.

Many practitioners have never had to learn even rudimentary verbal defensive skills in outside practice. Some have just said yes to any requests their patients made, so there was no need for confrontation. And if things got too uncomfortable, they could always just fire the patient! However, in corrections we have to say no, and we can't fire our patients. So learning to deal with verbal confrontations and manipulation is an essential correctional medicine skill. Without it practitioners will flounder, be unhappy, and quit.

Our Patients Don't Go Home

The final major difference between correctional medicine and medicine in the outside world is that our patients do not go home. We have a captive audience, literally! Believe it or not, this is a very important medical point.

Back in my previous life as an ER doc, if I asked a patient to come back tomorrow to be rechecked, I knew few of them would. It was just too much hassle. They had to find a ride back to the ER (especially hard for the homeless or those without cars), they had to endure another prolonged wait in the ER waiting room, and they would be charged big bucks for another ER visit—no wonder so few scheduled follow-ups actually returned!

Once I began to practice in a jail clinic, I realized the situation is much different. The patient I see in clinic today will not go home. She will go to her housing dorm down the hall. I know exactly where she will be tomorrow or in a week. If I want to see her again tomorrow, I can. In fact, I can reliably see her for follow-up anytime I want to.

You might think, *So what? What difference can it possibly make to the practice of medicine that our patients don't go home?* It does indeed have several important consequences. I can think of at least four.

1. *The eight-hour test*

Since I can see any patient back any time I want, I can easily do much more frequent checkups than I could in the ER. Consider a random patient I've evaluated in the ER for abdominal pain. Based on just their history and physical exam, I'm pretty sure there's no emergency here and this patient does not need to be admitted. But *pretty sure* is not the same as 100% sure. I would really like for him to be rechecked tomorrow. I'm afraid, though, that he won't come back tomorrow, for any or all the reasons mentioned above. Once I let him out of my sight, I probably will never see him again.

So instead of sending him home with a plan to recheck in 24 hours, instead I (and my ER colleagues) would do "the ER thing": tests, x-rays, and labs. We know most of these are of questionable value. But ordering them has one important benefit: It keeps the patient in the ER for several hours! That way I can recheck him to see how his condition changes over time.

In corrections I can do things quite differently. I don't have to order labs, x-rays, and tests to keep a patient around for serial examinations. I know exactly where he's going to be. I can arrange for him to be reevaluated in eight hours, 24 hours, or whenever I want! I can have the jail nurse check on him hourly, even, and call me with vital signs. I can bring him back to the clinic tomorrow or in a week. And I know it will happen!

I call this concept "the eight-hour test," and I've discovered it to be an essential medical test. I now use it all the time. It's a true medical test; the objective is to evaluate how the patient's condition changes over time. And it will reliably change. In eight hours patients will either be improved or worse. Either result tells me a lot about their condition! Being able to reliably do a time test makes me more confident about what's going on and less likely to order meaningless tests.

2. *Are patients regularly checked on?*

Occasionally there is a story in my local paper about someone found several days after they died. These patients typically lived alone or were homeless and had no one to check on them. Fear of this happening is what drives the thriving home monitor industry: "Help! I've fallen, and I can't get up!"

We don't have to worry about this in jails and prisons. Our patients are checked on daily by a variety of personnel. Patients who take medications are seen every day during med pass. Correctional personnel check on correctional patients daily during head counts, at recreation, and during meals.

I've lost count of the times some jail deputy has alerted me to a medical problem by saying, "You ought to see this guy—he doesn't look too good!"

It is not uncommon that the sickest patients won't put in a "kite" (a formal request for help) or complain. Thank goodness for the jail deputies who look out for them!

Not only that, but patients are available for their routine screening exams. It is very common in outside practice to "lose" patients. They just stop coming in for their appointments. Most of the time the doctor doesn't know why. Did they move? Die? Find a different practitioner? Or just decide going to the doctor for checkups was a hassle?

This does not happen in corrections. Even if the jail patient has forgotten their clinic appointment, someone will remind them. And why not go to scheduled checkups? It's not that much trouble—and what else is there to do? Of course, some people do refuse to be followed in chronic care clinics, but this is uncommon.

The result of this is that prisons routinely achieve medical goals outside clinics can't. Take the goal of getting diabetics' A1C levels below 8, for example. A typical outside primary care practice can expect 50% of its patients to achieve that goal. But prisons typically set (and achieve) 90% compliance.

3.   *We can observe patients in their "natural habitat."*

One of my jail patients once hobbled into my clinic and said his chronic back pain was so bad, he could barely get out of bed to eat. In fact, he struggled mightily to even get up from the waiting room chair. He insisted the only solution was for me to prescribe oxycodone, just like his outside doctor. He seemed to be in tremendous pain. But somehow, something didn't add up in my mind. I was suspicious. So I strolled down to the housing dorm to see for myself just how disabled this patient was. As it turned out, he was at rec playing—yes, you guessed it—basketball! I arrived just in time to see my patient execute a perfect reverse layup! True story.

Contrast this with outside doctors who have no way to verify the stories told to them. If a patient says he cannot play golf anymore, is that literally true? An orthopedist friend once told me about a patient who reported his back pain was so severe that he could no longer play golf. The orthopedist increased his pain prescription and scheduled an MRI.

The Best of Jail Medicine

However, the very next day he read in the paper that this patient was doing very well in his weekly golf league.

If a patient says she follows her diabetic diet strictly, does she really? My friend the endocrinologist had a diabetic patient whose A1C had significantly worsened since it was last checked six months earlier. Also, the patient had gained 12 pounds. "Are you sticking to your diabetic diet?" "Absolutely!" said the patient. "I never cheat."

We don't have this problem in jails and prisons. We can easily get details about our patients' behavior. If our patients tell us they're having trouble walking, we can observe them in the dorms to see how well they move. If a patient is not meeting his diabetic goal, we can check his commissary purchases. We can even see how compliant our patients are taking their prescribed medications simply by checking the medication administration record.

4. *We get to see the progression of disease.*

I am continually amazed at the medical pathology I see in jails and prisons. I often am literally the first doctor many jail patients have seen in years. Here is a typical encounter: "Hi, doc. I've had this bump on my arm for a long time." Jail doc: "Well, that's a cancer." Like a homeless clinic in a big city, jail medicine affords a practitioner the unique opportunity to see lots of neglected medical pathology.

Prison practitioners have noticed a similar phenomenon. It seems there are more interesting and rare diseases in our prisons than there are outside the walls. There is no research into this phenomenon I'm aware of, but I have talked to many physicians who believe it's true. Docs who have spent 25 years practicing internal medicine and then come to corrections say there's a much higher incidence of interesting, unusual, and downright rare medical conditions in prison medical practice.

Some have opined this could be due to the less-than-healthy lifestyles many led prior to coming to prison. I personally think a different factor is in play. I think this phenomenon is related to the fact that our patients don't leave our practices.

Consider the hypothetical case of Dr. Smith, a community family practitioner, who has a patient we'll call Joe. Dr. Smith has taken care of

Joe for 20 years. During that time Joe has had some mundane, routine accidents, hypertension, and other sorts of things followed by primary care. One day, though, Joe is discovered to have a rare case of metastatic cancer. What is likely to happen next is this: Joe will become the patient of his oncologist, cancer surgeon, and radiation oncologists. The oncologists follow him in clinics and hospital admissions. They are whom Joe calls when he has a problem. He may never see Dr. Smith again! But even if he does, it will be infrequently. Joe has essentially left the practice of Dr. Smith and become a patient of the specialists.

This happens over and over again with all sorts of unusual disease processes. Once patients develop something big, they are primarily followed by the appropriate specialist, whether a rheumatologist, neurologist, or whatever. Their original primary care doctor will see them rarely.

But this does not happen in prisons. Our patients with unusual and complex disease processes remain our patients. Sure, they'll go out to see the specialist, but they always return to us. We are the ones who implement the treatments, prescriptions, and recommendations of the specialists. We continue to see them in routine clinics for years. We see them before, during, and after radiation therapy. We watch them recover from surgery. We see what happens when, say, the rheumatologists try a novel drug.

This is the real reason there is so much more pathology in prisons than in outside primary care practices: Our patients do not leave. If you are a young physician who really wants to learn—to see a broad array of diseases and observe their progression—there are two places where you can get this experience: You can go to a third-world country, or you can practice in a prison.

I think this is a big selling point of correctional medicine that we have mostly failed to communicate to new recruits. There is no question, the fact that our patients do not go home has a big impact on our medical practice. This is one of the reasons why correctional medicine is such an interesting and great career!

The Best of Jail Medicine

DON'T BE THE DECIDER

A reader of my JailMedicine blog once asked about a patient who always wanted to bargain. "Well, if you're not going to do anything, can I have an extra mat?" or "Can I have a bottom floor restriction?" or "Transfer me then!" or "Give me insoles," and other such requests. Denials only generated more requests in an endless cycle. They sought advice on how to handle it.

We'll talk more about manipulative techniques later, but bargaining is one. It is an important and commonly used manipulation. I have also run across it: "Well, if you won't give me tramadol, can I at least have Flexeril?" Often it comes with a promise: "If you give me the Flexeril, I won't bother you anymore."

The goal of verbal jiujitsu is to deflect and avoid any confrontation. To do that you must understand why the confrontation occurred. The root cause of the confrontation described here was that my reader had become the decider. To solve the problem, stop being the decider.

To understand how this works, consider a person buying a new car who wants to pay less than the sticker price. The salesperson wants to sell them the car for the sticker price. But as soon as they say they want to pay $500 less, the salesperson says, "I'll have to check with my manager." She then leaves and comes back with the decision, either yes or no. The salesperson is not the decider.

The decider is the entity authorized to give the patient whatever it is they want. Your bargaining patient has identified you as that decider. You have confirmed you are the decider by saying no to their requests for the transfer and a bottom floor restriction. Saying no implies you could have said yes if you'd wanted to. Once that has been established, the patient thinks all he has to do to is convince you to change your mind. He starts with bargaining but maybe then progresses to a grievance and then a board complaint, all in an attempt to force you, the decider, to change your mind.

Of course, you can't win no matter what you do, because if you give in, you have proven this type of bargaining works. As a result lots of jail patients will want to bargain with you. But if you hold the hard line and don't give in, you still have lost, because your relationship with your patient has now become adversarial, time-consuming, and stressful.

So what is the solution? The solution is for you stop being the decider! Instead, the decider is going to be either a policy or a committee to which you defer. Official policies work well for stuff like second-mattress requests and bottom-floor restrictions. Once your facility has adopted a guideline for bottom-floor restrictions, the bargaining conversation goes like this:

"Well, at least give me a bottom-floor restriction."

"I can't. There is a policy for those, and I have to follow it."

You're not the decider anymore—the policy is!

Committees should be the decider for patients demanding special drugs (like narcotics for chronic pain) or unusual procedures (like an MRI for minor knee injury). Then your answer again is not no but rather "I can't approve that." If you don't have a therapeutics committee set up at your facility yet, in the meantime say, "I'll have to talk that over with my medical director (or colleagues)." Then get back to the patient later with the message that *they* (the decider) said no.

WORDS MATTER

Words matter. What we write about our patients in our medical notes to a great degree reflects how we feel about them. Our words also mold our future relationships with our patients.

One good example cited by Jayshil Patel, MD, in a 2018 *JAMA* editorial is the common phrase *The patient was a poor historian.*[1] There may be many reasons why a patient is not able to answer our questions well, such as dementia, delirium, or psychosis. In fact, the inability to present a cogent narrative usually is an important symptom of an underlying condition. *Poor historian* does not reflect this fact. To the contrary, *poor historian* implies the patient is at fault for my poor documentation, not me! *Poor historian* leaves out that there are other ways for me to get a medical history (medical records, talking to family, etc.). *Poor historian* also implies the patient was deliberately not cooperative—even though I spent maybe two minutes attempting to get a history.

Many other common medical phrases also subtly disparage patients. Two good examples are the words *denies* and *admits*, as in, "The patient denies drinking" or "the patient admits to IV heroin use." The implication of these words is that we are engaged in something akin to a hostile cross-examination where I forced the patient to admit (against their will) to drinking and I really don't believe the patient who "denies" drug use. Words guide how we think about our patients, even on a subconscious basis. When I use these words, I am saying my patient and I are not on the same team.

In corrections, perhaps the single best example of a word that negatively influences our relationship with our patients is *inmate.*

I have reviewed hundreds of correctional patient charts, and I can confidently say *inmate* (or the abbreviation *I/M*) is used more than patient or the person's name in correctional medical records. Now, I understand that our patients are inmates by definition. I also understand that we learn from others to use *inmate* in our medical documentation, and it becomes habitual. No malice is usually intended!

However, *inmate* is usually inappropriate in correctional medical documentation (in my opinion). When incarcerated people are in our medical clinics, they are primarily patients. Yes, they are also incarcerated, but this is irrelevant to their relationship to us.

Consider the example of people committed to psychiatric facilities. They are also inmates (by definition), but the medical professionals in state psychiatric facilities do not use the word *inmate* in their documentation. They say *patient* or use the patient's name. So why do we?

The answer, I think, is that we picked up the term *inmate* (or its prison equivalent, *offender*) from our security colleagues. Security is an ever-present concern in jails and prisons in a way it is not in a psychiatric hospital. We have to go through security to get in and wait to be buzzed through clanging metal doors. We have correctional officers or deputies always about—and we rely on them. They are our colleagues. The deputies say *inmate,* so we historically have used the same term.

But our relationship with the people incarcerated in a jail is very different than the relationship deputies have with them. When incarcerated people are in our medical clinic, they have become our patients. Using the term *inmate* in our medical documentation misidentifies our relationship. When I used to work in both the ER and county jail, I commonly would see the same patients in both locales.

"When did you get out of jail?" I'd say at the ER. "Yesterday."
"When did you get rearrested?" I'd say to the same person at my next jail clinic. "Yesterday."

My relationship with that person was the same in both circumstances. They were not an inmate in one setting and a patient in another. In both places I was their doctor, and they were my patient.

The Best of Jail Medicine

In our medical documentation, let's please get rid of the terms *inmate* and *I/M*. Let's instead use names or the general term *patient*.

Reference

1. Patel JJ. The Things We Say. *JAMA*. 2018; 319(4): 341–2. doi:10.1001/jama.2017.20545

OPERATIONS

'I Came to See the Doctor'

What is wrong with this picture?

I have a sore throat, swollen lymph glands, and an intermittent fever that won't go away after three weeks. Also, I am very, very fatigued. I can hardly work. I make an appointment and go to my doctor's office, where I am seen by a nurse. His nametag says Jerry, LPN. *Jerry examines me, tells me I have strep throat (without testing), gives me a prescription for amoxicillin, and sends me on my way.*

"Wait," I say. "Don't I get to see the doctor? I came to see my doctor!"

"Oh, I called the doctor," Jerry says. "Also, the doctor wrote a protocol to tell me what to do when patients come in with sore throat."

"Great!" I say. "I'm going to rate this appointment as a 10 on your feedback card!"

I see at least three things wrong with this scenario.

1. I never saw a doctor! I came to see a doctor. Jerry says he called the doctor, but the doctor did not see me herself, so she had to rely on whatever Jerry told her (plus Jerry's sore throat protocol).

2. The diagnosis and treatment were probably wrong. It is unlikely I have strep throat. My symptoms suggest infectious mononucleosis, in which case the amoxicillin is going to give me a monster rash.

3. And yet I rated this experience highly. That's unlikely!

I think we all would agree this little vignette is not realistic. Medical encounters do not happen this way in the community. Patients would not rate such an experience highly and would instead stop going to a medical practice that operated this way. The practice would fail. When you go to a clinic, an emergency department, a "doc in the box," or your own doctor's office, you see the doctor.

We also would agree that my clinical scenario was bad medicine all the way around.

And yet this is exactly how many medical clinics operate in correctional medicine! I have seen systems set up this way to one degree or another in both prisons and jails, but the worst offenders seem to be smaller community jails.

Such jails have a medical system in which the primary medical care of acute complaints (like a sore throat) or even potentially life-threatening conditions (like alcohol withdrawal) is managed by nurses who rely on written protocols. The nurses may be RNs, but if RNs are too hard to recruit or too expensive, the jail nurse could instead be an LPN. Whichever nurse sees the patient for a sore throat or alcohol withdrawal may or may not call a physician, but even when they do, the physician does not always personally see the patient.

I realize it is not possible for the correctional physician to go into the jail each and every time a patient has a problem. This is especially true in jails where there's high turnover, and you don't know what medical problem is going to show up off the streets.

For example, if a nurse calls about a newly booked heroin addict with an infected injection site, I have no problem with starting an antibiotic and starting treatment for heroin withdrawal based on a written guideline. But the next time there's a jail practitioner clinic, that patient should be seen by the practitioner. This is how it should work on the outside as well.

The reasons why practitioners may think it is OK to diagnose and treat patients in jails without ever seeing them vary, but these come to mind.

1. Some doctors have their own busy practices and provide service to the jail on the side. They may even feel they are covering the jail more or less as a favor to the community.

2. Doctors often don't think of the incarcerated as "their" patients in the same way as patients in their regular practice.

3. They're just doing the same thing the last physician at the jail did. It's always been done this way!

4. Doctors may feel they don't get paid enough to spend more time physically present at the jail.

5. No one complains! The sheriff doesn't complain, jail patients don't complain, the community doesn't complain.

These reasons and others may allow physicians to feel remote diagnosis and treatment of incarcerated patients is perfectly fine. Personally, though, I strongly feel the people in my jails are my patients and should be treated the same as any other of my patients. That means seeing them each and every time I authorize an urgent prescription over the phone.

MEDICAL CLEARANCE

When arresting officers arrive with their charges at a certain large urban jail, the first person they see when they come through the doors is a nurse. The nurse quickly evaluates the arrested person to determine whether a medical clearance is needed before the person can be booked. If a clearance is needed, the arresting officer must transport the prisoner to a local ER and then return with the medical clearance in hand.

One evening (so the story goes) an arresting officer arrived at the jail bodily dragging a prisoner through the prebook door by the backseat of his pants and coat. "This guy's an asshole," the officer said. "He won't do anything I ask. He just ignores me." He then dumps the prisoner on the floor. The nurse kneels by the prisoner briefly, looks up, and says, "That's because he's dead!"

Medical clearances are a hugely important and often neglected part of the jail medical process.

Many people who are arrested need urgent medical attention before they're booked into jail. An easy example is the person arrested for drunk driving but who was seriously injured in the motor vehicle accident they caused. Another is the person who has a heart attack as they are being arrested. No one would disagree that it's wrong and cruel to take these people to jail for booking before they receive medical care.

The problem is that arresting officers often do not like to take the people they arrest to the ER for medical evaluation and clearance. Escorting these prisoners takes them out of service, sometimes for several hours. They complain that often the ER docs don't really do a real exam. They glance briefly at the patient and fill out the clearance form. The officers consider this to be a waste of time.

Everyone will agree, though, that there are some people who clearly belong in the hospital rather than jail—like the severely injured trauma victim. Others are not really sick and can be safely delivered to the jail, where they can be evaluated by the jail's medical team. The problem is that the decision as when to take an arrestee to the ER for medical clearance and when to go directly to jail must be made by a nonmedical person: the arresting officer. It would be helpful to them to have written guidance as to which prisoners need medical clearance and which do not.

It's important for arresting officers and jail personnel to understand there are three reasons for obtaining a medical clearance before taking a person to jail. The first is that it is best for the patient. Taking an arrested person with urgent medical needs directly to jail delays necessary medical care and can lead to bad outcomes. The difference between going directly to the ER and going to the jail first for processing and then to the ER can be hours. Sick patients can deteriorate rapidly in that time.

Second, going directly to the ER for medical clearance saves money because it is more efficient to get urgent medical care before booking. Third, the final reason to obtain medical care before booking is that this markedly decreases legal liability should a bad outcome occur. No one can always predict how sick an injured patient or patient with chest pain really is, especially if they are intoxicated or upset at being arrested. Obtaining a medical clearance before booking shows the arresting officer isn't being deliberately indifferent to a potentially serious medical need.

I would recommend every jail develop a guideline on which patients should be medically cleared before coming to jail and then set up a conference to discuss that guideline with all the arresting agencies that bring prisoners to the jail—city police, county deputies, state police, and probation and parole—as well as the jail's legal counsel. If all arresting agencies adopt the guidelines, this will absolutely improve medical care, decrease overall costs, and reduce legal risk for the jail.

Outside Physicians

Those of us who practice medicine in jails frequently (daily!) run into the thorny issue of our relationships with the doctors who care for our patients outside of jail.

When patients are in our jails, we are responsible for them; they are our patients. But these patients also have doctors outside of jail that they perhaps have been seeing for years. The jail patient considers their outside physician their "real" doctor, not us. (Throughout this article, I am going to use the term *doctors* rather than the more generic *practitioners*. I do not mean to slight nurse practitioners or physician assistants. What I say applies to them as well.)

A case occurred in one of my jails recently where a patient came to jail with prescriptions filled out by his outside physician that authorized him to have a double mattress, an extra blanket, and an extra pillow. (There was no note requiring us to feed him pizza every Friday night—he must have forgotten to ask for that.) So, I was left in a little dilemma. What should I do about these orders? Ignore them? Allow the patient to have the extra comfort items?

Dealing with incarcerated patients' outside physicians can be tricky, but I have found (mostly through sad experience) there are definitely right and wrong ways to handle these encounters. The right way involves recognizing three important points:

1. The outside physician is not authorized to write orders for patients in the jail. She does not have staff privileges in the jail setting.
2. Patients sometimes pit their outside doctors against jail doctors to get their way. It can be a form of manipulation.

3. The easiest and most time-effective way to defuse this situation is to speak to the outside physician directly and come to a joint decision about what will be done for the patient in jail.

Staff Privileges

The first core issue here that was misunderstood by both the patient and the outside physician is one of staff privileges. Just like hospitals, jails and prisons have staff privilege systems. If a patient of mine is admitted to the local hospital, I cannot write or call in orders. To do so I would have to formally apply for staff privileges at that hospital. Even then I could not write orders for patients at the hospital unless I was their admitting or attending physician. This staff privilege system is common to all medical establishments. I likewise cannot call in orders at the local nursing home or walk into the urgent care center across the street and start seeing patients.

It is the same at a jail or a prison. To practice medicine in a correctional facility, a physician must be granted staff privileges at that facility. Who grants these privileges? The person with legal authority to operate the facility. In the case of almost all jails, that would be the sheriff and jail administrator.

What this means, of course, is that I, as the medical director of the jail, have no obligation to honor any outside physician's orders. In fact, the outside physician cannot make orders—she has no staff privileges. If I or the other jail medical providers think an outside physician's recommendations are a good idea, we must rewrite their order; it must come from us. On the other hand, if I, in my professional judgment, think an order from an outside physician is inappropriate, I am under no obligation to follow it. I should, of course, document exactly why I made my decision so there is no question later.

But this does not solve the problem raised by this outside physician's orders and the patient's insistence that we follow them. What the patient is doing here is pitting two physicians against each other. This happens all the time in jail. Jail patients will say their outside physician has prescribed certain medical treatments. If I, as the jail physician, say no to these requests, the patient feels he has a legitimate grievance: "My outside doctor has prescribed *x,* and you won't let me have it. My outside doctor is my real doctor and knows me and my medical problems way better than you do."

The patient has become the spokesperson for the outside physician.

Direct Communication

By far the best way to deal with this problem is to call the outside physician by telephone and come to common ground. I have found this to be quite easy and pleasant for the most part. I have found outside physicians, for the most part, to be thoughtful, reasonable, and helpful.

So it was in this case. I called the outside physician and explained the jail policy about extra mattresses and other comfort requests. She admitted she didn't know much about jail medical procedures and had written that note only because the patient begged her to. I asked if she would support me in my determination of appropriate housing for this patient's medical condition, and of course she agreed. By the end of the conversation, we were chatting like old comrades. I gave her my personal cell phone number in case she had any questions about future patients who might end up in jail.

And finally I could report to the patient that I had personally talked to his outside physician, we had jointly developed a housing and treatment plan for him while he was in jail, and this would not include an extra blanket, extra mattress, or extra pillow. Problem solved. He is no longer able to play one doctor versus another.

Added Benefits

There are lots of added benefits to calling the outside physician in cases like this. It consumes much less time than fighting with the patient over the course of several clinic visits and grievances. It develops personal contacts in the outside medical community. If I have a question in this doctor's field, now I can call her for help. The doctor also knows more about the jail and jail medicine than she did before. We have a rapport that will come in handy the next time one of her patients ends up in jail. The next time one of her patients asks her to authorize special treatment in jail, she will know not to do this (or at least to call me first).

Note that requesting medical records would not have achieved the same results. In fact, requesting medical records would have accomplished nothing and wasted time. The act of calling and speaking personally to the outside physician is the key.

As usual, this strategy worked wonderfully in this case. Once I told the patient his outside doctor and I agreed on the treatment he would receive in jail, he had nothing further to say. He never brought the subject up again. He never wrote a grievance.

MEDICAL NECESSITY

Modern medicine is miraculous in ways both big and small. I have seen big miracles in my jail patients—lives saved from cancer and heart disease and hepatitis, patients who would have died due to these conditions 20 years ago. I, myself have not yet had any big medical problems like these (knock on wood), but I have experienced several smaller miracles of modern medicine, each of which has immeasurably improved my life. I would like to share four of these.

Several years ago I developed persistent pain in my left shoulder. I thought it was a tendinitis due to exercise and tried to decrease shoulder-intensive exercises. The pain worsened. My shoulder hurt all day but especially ached at night. I was waking up every night due to shoulder pain. I tried sleeping in different positions to see if one was better. I tried various methods of taping the shoulder. And I took lots of NSAIDs. But nothing helped. You should understand that the pain was never debilitating; I never missed work. I never even stopped exercising. But I lived with constant low-level pain every minute of every day and night for almost a year.

Eventually an MRI showed I had a large tear of the rotator cuff and impingement syndrome caused by a narrow subacromial space. An orthopedist took me to surgery and did a repair.

I remember waking up in the recovery room—and for the first time in a year, my shoulder didn't hurt! Except for the pain of rehab, my shoulder has not hurt—at all—ever since. I cannot describe how great a blessing this has been for my quality of life! It was an amazing thing. I certainly didn't wait very long to get my other shoulder fixed when the same problems developed there.

My hernia surgery was similar. I had small bilateral hernias that didn't bother me too much. My friend the surgeon told me not to wait too long to get them repaired because the smaller they are, the easier they are to fix. But I waited about nine months. Over that period the hernias definitely got bigger. Fortunately they were still small enough that the repair was easy. I was back to work in just a couple of days.

For years I struggled with painful cracks on my heels. My solution was to superglue them, but despite this my dry, cracked heels were a constant low-level irritation. Then I discovered over-the-counter Aquaphor, which is similar to Vaseline. Since I began applying Aquaphor to my heels every day underneath my socks, I have never had another painful heel crack. How could I have not known about this for so long? Amazing!

Finally, a relatively new drug on the market is diclofenac gel. This is wonderful stuff! It works far better than oral NSAIDs or Tylenol for arthritis pain I get in my hands and tendinitis I get in my elbows and heels from time to time. Since I discovered diclofenac gel, I have nearly stopped taking ibuprofen altogether! Very cool!

What does all this have to do with correctional medicine? Well, each of these four medical treatments that have immeasurably improved my quality of life may be denied to incarcerated patients as not being "medically necessary." Had I been incarcerated, I likely would never have had shoulder surgery approved, since I had no functional disability. I might not have been approved for hernia surgery for years, until the hernias were much bigger and problematic (and, by the way, much harder to repair). Many correctional facilities, especially jails, do not allow patients access to skin moisturizers like Aquaphor. Diclofenac gel is not on many correctional formularies (though this may change since it is becoming inexpensive).

What does the term *medically necessary* mean? I understand the need to operate within a budget (however arbitrary). I understand that sometimes medical care can impact the security of a correctional facility. And I understand that incarcerated people, kind of by definition, do not have access to everything available on the outside.

But I have practiced correctional medicine for years in both jails and prisons, and if I have learned anything, I have learned this: The issue of what *medically necessary* means lies at the heart of our profession. Is a rotator cuff repair medically necessary? Early hernia surgery? Aquaphor? Diclofenac gel? All of these are debatable. Smart and caring correctional physicians whom I respect may disagree with me. But personally I don't see how I can ethically deny my correctional patients access to the medical procedures and treatments that have been the most important in my own life.

THE COMPLIANCE TRAP

I had a patient recently who demonstrated what I call the "compliance trap" of corrections. The compliance trap is simply this: Outside jail, in the real world, most people do not take their medications perfectly. They miss doses. They forget sometimes. Many studies have demonstrated this. But when these same people come to jail, they get their medications passed to them every dose—they don't miss doses. They are compliant with their medication dosing in a way they weren't on the outside. And this can sometimes get them into trouble.

Take, for example, the patient who came to my jail with a prescription for 600 mg of Dilantin a day. This is a huge dose! But he had a legitimate prescription for it, and so it was continued at the same dose in jail. However, two weeks later he began to have nausea, vomiting, and dizziness. We checked his Dilantin level, and he was toxic! His dose of 600 mg a day was, indeed, too big for this patient. In fact, after we adjusted his dose and checked his levels a couple of times, we found the proper dose for this patient was a more modest 400 mg a day.

How did this happen? I did not interrogate this patient's outside doctor, but I think I know what happened. He kept returning to the outside clinic with subtherapeutic blood levels of Dilantin, and the doctor kept increasing the dose. However, the reason the patient had subtherapeutic blood levels was not that he was a superrapid metabolizer of Dilantin; rather, he just hadn't been taking it every day. He'd been missing doses.

But when he came to jail, the jail nurses made sure he didn't miss any doses, and quickly he was toxic.

So that is the compliance trap. Outside of jail many patients do not take their medications regularly or at all. When they come to jail, they don't miss doses. And sometimes this can make them sick.

Dilantin is one example, but there are several more. All of these are real examples from my jails. Do any sound familiar?

- A small (110-pound) woman takes six lithium 300 mg tablets a day.
- A man with deep vein thrombosis takes 15 mg of Coumadin a day.
- A woman with bipolar disorder takes 1,500 mg of Depakote a day.

Now, perhaps these are all legitimate doses, carefully titrated based on perfectly compliant patients. However, you could also easily fall into the compliance trap and end up with a toxic patient. The only way to know is to check appropriate monitoring levels a week, say, after they arrive in the jail.

(By the way, one of the three examples above turned out to be a proper, legitimate prescription based on blood levels. I'll leave it to you to guess which one!)

An interesting variation of the compliance trap has to do with insulin doses. Believe it or not, some patients with diabetes are not compliant with their diabetic diets outside jail. They eat at Burger King, McDonald's, and Pizza Hut—all in the same day! They raid their refrigerator for chocolate ice cream at 2 a.m. The amount of insulin they use is dosed accordingly.

Once they come to jail and all they get to eat is a proper diabetic diet, their outside insulin dose is suddenly way too much, and they get hypoglycemic.

Another interesting variation of the compliance trap is posed by methamphetamine abusers. Many of them are also psychiatric patients being prescribed sedating psych meds like Seroquel, trazodone, and Ambien by their psychiatry providers (who, of course, do not know they are doing meth). When they come to jail and no longer have access to meth, their sedating medications are now no longer counterbalanced by amphetamines, and they become overly sedated.

Keep the compliance trap in mind, especially when patients present with big doses of meds. It may save you a lot of grief!

Utilization Management Is Different in Corrections

This is an important fact I have learned from many years working in prisons and jails: Most correctional practitioners do not understand how utilization management in a prison system works. They misunderstand what the goal of the UM process is. They misunderstand the process of submitting requests. And they misunderstand how decisions are made. It took me a full three years of working in a prison system before I wrapped my head around how UM is supposed to function. This is because UM within a correctional system is fundamentally different than UM in the outside world. As well, new incoming correctional practitioners are not taught how prison UM works or how to make UM requests properly.

To show how utilization management in a prison is different than with a typical health maintenance organization (HMO) in the outside world, let's say I am a primary care practitioner in the community who wants to order an MRI on one of my patients. As we all know from long experience, I can't just order the MRI. I have to get it *preauthorized*. To do that I have to submit paperwork to the patient's insurance company explaining why I want to do the procedure. Someone will review my request, but I will have no idea who this person is or what their qualifications are. The reviewer could be a physician, or it could be a nurse referring to UM guidelines. I don't know and never will. Whoever that person is, they will either approve payment for the procedure or deny it.

Notice several important things about this interaction:

1. I do not know the person reviewing the request I sent in. They do not know me.

2. If the UM reviewer denies the request, that doesn't mean I can't do the procedure—it just means the insurance company won't pay for it. The

patient can still have the procedure done if they want to pay for it out of their own pocket.

3. If I disagree with a UM denial, I cannot pick up a phone and call the individual who made that decision to ask, "What were you thinking?" Instead I would have to write a formal appeal. In fact, all communications in a typical HMO must be formally written.

4. The UM reviewer (whoever that might be) does not comment on my case other than to approve or deny the request I made. They never say, for example, "What are *you* thinking? Read the literature! Instead of ordering an MRI, you ought to do a CT!" Utilization management within an HMO is not a friendly collaboration between colleagues. Instead it is an impersonal request for *payment*. It's as impersonal as using PayPal for an online purchase.

Now consider the identical case within a prison. I'm still asking for the same MRI. Even though the prison process is called by the same name as in an HMO—*utilization management*—correctional UM is an entirely different animal. First, if I again am the primary care practitioner at the site requesting an MRI, I know the physician who's going to review my request. We probably communicate all the time in other matters, such as committee meetings, site visits, etc. Shoot, we may have had beers together after a conference!

Second, I know the physician who reviews the case will not simply "deny" the request. If she does not approve the request, she must instead send back an alternative treatment plan (ATP) that describes what she thinks I should do instead of an MRI. In other words, the process has become a discussion about the proper care to be provided to this patient. We are, in fact, collaborating.

As I mentioned before, there is no collaboration in an HMO. There is only an impersonal yes-or-no question of payment. By contrast, in a prison I am really asking my colleague, "What do you think about his case? Should I do an MRI?" The answer could be, "Great idea! Go ahead." The answer could also be, "I don't think so. Here are my thoughts in an alternative treatment plan. Let's talk about this case."

At this point the question is how to continue the discussion. In an HMO, if I want to appeal a denial, I will have to write a formal appeal. And the only answer I can expect is another *approved* or *denied* answer. In a prison, again, everything is different. The person who sent me the ATP is my colleague. What is the best way to communicate with her?

Unfortunately, prison UM systems are sometimes based on the HMO model, and primary care practitioners are expected to write formal appeals just as they would on the outside. In my opinion this is crazy! This is my colleague, not an unknown bureaucrat. The best way to communicate with a colleague in the modern world is *not* via letter! The best way to collaborate on this case would be to pick up a telephone! Alternatively, I could send an email, write a text, or walk down the hall to her office. Any of these will be faster and more efficient than writing out an appeal form.

It's just a short distance from this to the next insight into prison utilization management: If I know a request for an MRI has to go through the UM system and will be reviewed there by my colleague, why not pick up the phone and discuss the case with her *before* I fill out the initial UM form? This will save time if my request will eventually be denied, since I won't have to fill out all the paperwork. It will even save time if my request will be approved. Talking is simply the most efficient way to communicate with someone I know well.

So why don't prison practitioners do it this way? The answer is simple: They all came to prison medicine from the outside and are familiar and practiced in how UM works in HMOs. No one has pointed out how different things are in prisons. We should change this.

Patient Satisfaction

I think we'd all agree that in the wide world of medicine outside of jails and prisons, patient satisfaction is critically important. This is partly because patients are not just patients, they are also business clients. If they aren't happy, they'll go to some other doctor and hospital. Many studies have shown that patient satisfaction scores correlate strongly to revenue and market share. That is why hospitals routinely track patient satisfaction scores. Studies have also shown that roughly 80% of patient complaints are generated by fewer than 10% of practitioners. These complaint-prone physicians, PAs, and NPs are often "shown the door" by hospitals and practice groups. Their negative impact on revenue is just too great to ignore, even if they otherwise practice good medicine.

But, as I have often heard, correctional medicine is different. Our patients are a captive group (literally!). They cannot go to a different practitioner if they are unhappy. We do not have to please our patients to stay in business. Our "market share" does not rely on patient satisfaction. Plus, because of safety and security issues, we have to say no to patient requests more than outside physicians; and of course incarcerated patients are not going to be happy about that. So who cares if jail patients are unsatisfied?

The answer is we all should care. A lot.

There are two main reasons for this. First is the time-management issue. Jail patients unhappy with their medical care may not be able to leave, but they certainly can return time and again to the clinic, write grievances, complain to their families, and contact the ACLU. Responding to these efforts takes time. In the end it takes less time and effort to develop a trusting patient relationship than it does to respond to complaints and grievances.

Second (and more important), it is hard to practice good medicine if your patient does not trust you. The medical efficacy of everything we do is enhanced if the patient trusts us and believes in us. On the other hand, our medical efficacy is hindered if our patients question our competence or sincerity. Even in corrections we want and need our patients to be happy with their medical care.

However, this can be harder for us in corrections to accomplish than it is for outside practitioners. Our patients come into our facilities already mistrusting the "system," which includes us. Many patients, maybe even most, start out not believing we have their welfare at heart. We truly do have to say no to patient requests more than outside doctors, so we often start out fighting an uphill battle in gaining their trust. This makes it even more important to pay attention to factors that engender trust with our patients. But what are those factors?

Interestingly, there is a surprising amount of published literature addressing the question of what patients like and dislike in their interactions with practitioners. My favorite CME site, Primary Care Medical Abstracts, recently published 51 such articles—51! Who knew that much research existed? I would like to summarize what these articles said.

Patients want their doctors to look like doctors.

This is not so surprising. All of us, including you and me, tend to make initial judgments of competence by appearance. What would you think if the pilot of your next airline flight sauntered on board looking like the lead singer of a rock-and-roll hair band? Patients are no different. In studies people were shown pictures of doctors and asked which doctor they would prefer. Not surprisingly, they wanted their doctor to look like doctors. They liked white coats. They liked nice shirts, nice pants, nice shoes. They liked cleanliness. They did not like sandals, t-shirts, or jeans. They did not like provocative clothing—no miniskirts, cleavage, or muscle shirts. They didn't like earrings on men or gaudy jewelry on women. Interestingly, they didn't care one way or another about ties. And they thought scrubs were OK. The more a doctor's appearance deviated from the test subjects' perception of what a doctor should look like, the more the subjects questioned their competence.

(Note: Sometimes I will use the term doctors *and sometimes* practitioners. *I mean to include with both terms physicians, physician assistants, and nurse practitioners. This particular study asked test subjects about doctors, but the answers would not have changed for any medical practitioner. Actually, the principles I discuss here would equally apply to nurses in their encounters with patients as well).*

Of course, you don't *have to* dress professionally to do your job. But if you don't look like a professional, you will constantly have to overcome the instinctive perception that you're not a very good doctor. And remember: We in corrections already start out being mistrusted.

Patients want their clinics to be clean.

I've seen this slip in correctional facilities. But again, medical professionals are partly judged on our competence by how clean our clinics are. I recently toured the DeBerry Special Needs Facility in Nashville. The warden there, Bruce Westbrooks, talked about his belief that facility cleanliness is the basic key to every other part of prison discipline. If a prison facility is clean and well-maintained, he said, there are fewer fights, fewer rule violations, etc. Once cleanliness slips, this is perceived by both patients and staff as a lax attitude toward discipline in general, and as a result everything else slips with time.

I agree with Westbrooks and believe this is even more important in a healthcare setting. Patients, including patients, expect clinics to look and smell clean. If one doesn't, they will immediately suspect lack of caring and competence by the staff.

Patients want their doctors to be attentive and listen.

Here is an interesting study: Doctor No. 1 walked into an ER patient's room and did a quick history and physical. Doctor No. 2 did exactly the same thing. The only difference was that doctor No. 1 stood up during the whole exchange, and doctor No. 2 sat down. Patients were then asked how long the doctor spent talking to them.

I found this amazing: When the doctor sat down, patients perceived he spent *twice as much time* with them, even though the two doctors spent exactly the same amount of time in the room. The teaching point here is that we communicate with our patients in many nonverbal ways. Standing gives the impression that "I am in a hurry to get out of here." Sitting gives the impression that "I am settling in so I can listen." Other nonverbal cues patients like are when the doctor looks them in the eye and nods to show they are listening. Such behaviors are habits that take no extra time but result in increased patient satisfaction.

Another good habit is to allow the patient to speak without interruption and then state back to them what their complaint is. Doctors are notorious for interrupting patients too quickly. I, myself have this bad habit, but I have found that if I can stifle myself and let the patient talk, the better *and faster* the clinic visit usually goes. I've found patients themselves will give me the signal that they're ready for me to chime in by pausing and looking for a response. The difference in time between when I (in my impatience) would have interrupted them and when they give the "pause" signal is generally less than 30 seconds.

Patients like their doctors to explain things.

This is a concept practitioners commonly misunderstand. As an example, one study looked at patients who went to an urgent care center expecting to be prescribed an antibiotic. After the clinic visit the patients were asked to rate their satisfaction with it. Who do you think tended to be happier with the visit, those who got the antibiotic they expected or those who did not? The surprising answer was those who did not! Why? Because the practitioners who did not prescribe the antibiotic had to explain why! The ones who gave the antibiotic prescriptions just wrote them and handed them over without talking much. The key satisfaction factor here was whether the practitioner talked to the patient and explained things!

Incarcerated patients are no different. We correctional practitioners often have to say no to patient requests. If we explain why we're doing things differently than the patient expects, this goes a long way to assuage their disappointment. Many will actually leave the clinic satisfied.

I have also found it important to explain the natural course of the patient's condition. For example, people with coughs from chest colds need to know these coughs often persist for a long time, sometimes more than a month. If you don't explain this, they are going to be back in your clinic in a week complaining, "I'm no better." Same thing with tendonitis

The Best of Jail Medicine

and other musculoskeletal "tweaks." These do not get better quickly. Other conditions, like simple UTIs in healthy women, should be all the way better in two days after you give antibiotics. If they are not better by then, patients need to know to come back.

Patients like to know how long they're going to wait.

These studies were done in hospital ER waiting rooms. Surprisingly, satisfaction scores did not relate well to overall waiting time. People know when they go to an ER that they are going to have to wait. Rather, satisfaction scores were related to whether their expectations of *how long the wait would be* were met. For example, if patients were told the wait would be one hour and they waited less than an hour, they were happy. But if they waited more than an hour, they were unhappy. The expectation was set when they were told how long the wait would be. Patients also were unhappy if others in the waiting room "jumped ahead" and were called before them.

In corrections, one "wait" is the time from when a patient submits a nonemergency medical request until they are seen in clinic. Another is the time from when we draw labs or do x-rays until we inform the patient of the results. Here is the key concept: We set the patients' expectation when we tell them how long this wait will be.

Let's say, for example, the average time it takes to get an x-ray report back from a radiologist and schedule a follow-up appointment is three days. If we tell patients we'll let them know x-ray results "in a couple of days" but they wait three, the patients will be unhappy and complain. This is just human nature. Instead, it is better to overestimate the wait time so you always meet the expectation! Instead of saying "a couple of days," tell them about a week. Then, when the appointment happens in three days, the patient will be happy you were so quick!

The take-home message from these 51 articles is that by changing how we interact with our patients in simple ways, we can markedly improve their satisfaction with our care, reduce complaints and grievances, and generally make life better for everyone. Try this experiment: Pick one or two ways in which you can improve your interactions with patients— dressing better, cleaning the clinic, better eye contact, etc. I bet you'll notice an improvement in patient demeanor within a week.

GRIEVANCE RESPONSES

Benjamin Franklin once famously quipped, "Nothing is certain but death and taxes." However, Franklin didn't work in a jail. Otherwise he would have said, "Nothing is certain except death, taxes, and grievances."

On the outside patients don't write grievances—they vote with their feet. If they dislike the medical care they're receiving, they'll just go to a different doctor. In a jail they can't do this. We have a grievance system in correctional medicine because our patients can't fire us (and we can't fire them). If jail patients are unhappy with their medical care, their only recourse is to write a grievance.

Grievances aren't necessarily bad things. A medical grievance is sometimes the way by which jail patients alert us to mistakes we made or significant problems we may not have known about. I have had my butt saved in this manner more than once! Many grievances are simply about communication errors, where we have not yet adequately explained a medical decision to the patient.

Yet jail medical personnel often have a bad attitude about grievances. This is unfortunate because medical grievances are an important—even essential—part of the jail medical system. I believe the most important reason for the bad attitude is that jail medicine practitioners haven't been taught how to write a proper grievance response.

Stripped of all its emotional overlay, the grievance is a simple question about medical care. However, since this question is often accompanied by angry and demanding language, it tends to elicit angry and defensive emotions. To write a good grievance response, it is important to get past this emotional component and just focus on the question being asked. If this is done well, the patient will feel understood, and even if they don't receive what they want, the matter will be resolved. Do this poorly, and the patient will be even more hostile and plan their next move. The matter is not resolved and will have to be readdressed later.

It is also important to remember the grievance response may later be read by a patient advocate, such as a plaintiff's attorney or the ACLU. A poorly written grievance response may suggest you're denying reasonable medical care and have a bad attitude to boot. A good grievance response will show the patient's question was thoughtfully addressed, and no essential care was denied.

Who should write the grievance response?

The first question to consider is who should answer the grievance. Initial grievances should be answered by the medical person with greatest knowledge about the question being posed. A grievance relating to nursing care ("I wasn't offered my medications this morning!") should be answered by a nurse. This may be the director of nursing or another nurse assigned by the director. Similarly, dental complaints should be answered by the dentist, mental health complaints by mental health staff, and grievances about medical care by a practitioner, usually assigned by the medical director.

One question that often comes up is that if the grievance is about a specific person ("Nurse Joan was rude to me!"), should that person (Nurse Joan) or someone else respond? My feeling is that it should be someone else. Otherwise it puts Nurse Joan in the position of either arguing ("No, I wasn't! You were rude to me!") or feeling like she has to apologize even if she felt she did nothing wrong. It is better in my book to have someone else evaluate the complaint and write the response.

What if the patient appeals the response? Grievance-response appeals should be answered by a different person with equal or higher authority. For example, if a nurse answered the first grievance, the director of nursing could answer an appeal. The medical director of the facility can answer any type of appeal, whether nursing, dental, or mental health. In some cases the jail commander should be the person to answer a medical grievance or appeal, especially if the grievance is abusive.

What's the time frame for grievance responses?

In my opinion grievance responses should be written as soon as possible, certainly no more than a week after the grievance is received. An immediate response tells the patient you're taking their concerns seriously and care about your reply. Waiting a long time to respond tells the patient they're not important and gives them time to get angrier and maybe write other letters of complaint. It is always in our best interest—as well as the best interest of the patient—to respond quickly. In my grievance replies I list the date the date the grievance was written (or the date I received it, if it sat on someone's desk for a while): *"This is a response to a grievance dated January 25, 2019 and received by me January 30, 2019."*

How to Write a Grievance Reply

This is how I personally respond to grievances.

Step 1: Start with the essential information.

Grievance replies don't have to be formal letters but do need to include the basics: the date, the facility, what patient wrote the grievance and when, who is writing the response, and the fact this is a grievance response.

Date: 1/25/2019

Facility: Nurmengard Correctional Facility

"This is a response to a grievance written by Tom Marvolo Riddle, dated 1/24/2019."

Step 2: Restate the question.

The first sentence of the grievance response should restate the question being asked. Again, it is important to avoid reacting to or using emotional language. I prefer to write grievance replies in the third person—it feels more detached and less argumentative (though others disagree and feel the grievance reply should address the patient in the first person).

"In this grievance Mr. Riddle states he asked for a second mattress and this request was denied."

Sometimes it works to quote what the patient stated in their grievance directly.

"Mr. Riddle states, 'I am being denied medical treatment for my chronic pain.'"

Step 3: Explain what you did to evaluate the grievance.

After restating the complaint, the next step is to list all the things you did to investigate its validity. This includes the materials you reviewed (like medical records), the people you talked to, and the research you did. This is important because it shows that you took the grievance seriously by looking at all aspects of the complaint.

"I have reviewed Mr. Riddle's medical record, talked to the practitioner involved, and reviewed medical records from Mr. Riddle's outside medical provider."

Step 4: State your conclusion.

In my opinion this should not be a long, detailed rebuttal. This should be a short summary of your conclusion—1–2 sentences at most. You can offer to go into more detail about this issue in the next step.

"As was discussed with Mr. Riddle during his clinic visit, a second mattress is not a medical device or prescription. His outside medical records do not show any mention or order for medical bedding. This is not a medical issue."

"I have discussed Mr. Riddle's case directly with his outside pain management specialist, Dr. Pomfrey. We are in agreement about the care to be provided while Mr. Riddle is incarcerated."

Step 5: Offer to discuss the issue in more detail in medical clinic.

"Mr. Riddle may certainly discuss this issue in more detail in medical clinic if he wishes."

"I note Mr. Riddle is already scheduled be seen in the medical clinic, where we can discuss the case in more detail."

What if the patient is right?

In my experience medical grievances often have merit in whole or part. When this is the case, we should admit this, thank the patient for bringing it to our attention, and say what we're going to do to remedy the situation.

"Mr. Riddle states he is supposed to be taking buspirone twice a day, but since he arrived at the jail, it has only been dispensed once a day. I have reviewed the medical record and note Mr. Riddle is correct. I will rewrite the order for twice a day and ensure it is on the cart twice a day. I will also talk to Mr. Riddle directly in medical clinic."

What if the patient is abusing the grievance system?

Patients sometimes cross the line into unacceptable behavior in their grievances. Examples include using unacceptable language, calling medical providers names, and writing repetitive or trivial grievances. These usually should be given to the jail commander, who can both reply and decide on appropriate discipline.

Putting It All Together: An Example Grievance Response

Patient: Barty Crouch Jr.

Jail: Nurmengard Correctional Facility

Date: 2/13/2018

"This is a response to a grievance dated 2/12/18 in which Mr. Crouch states his complaint of rectal bleeding has not been adequately evaluated by medical services. I have reviewed his medical record and spoken to the practitioners who saw Mr. Crouch. I note that Mr. Crouch was seen for this complaint originally on 1/8/18 and had a normal rectal exam with no blood found by chemical testing. Mr. Crouch was scheduled for routine follow-up in the medical clinic on 1/22/18 and denied at that visit that he was still having rectal bleeding. Mr. Crouch has submitted no requests to be seen by medical since then. It appears to me Mr. Crouch has been appropriately assessed for his original complaint. However, since Mr. Crouch's symptoms have returned, I have scheduled him to be reevaluated at the next medical clinic."

How to Write an Alternative Treatment Plan

Many of us in supervisory positions in correctional medicine have utilization management (UM) duties. One common duty is to review requests from primary care practitioners for patient care procedures like referrals or, say, an MRI. We must then decide whether to approve the request or write an alternative treatment plan (ATP). This process is loosely based on a similar practice done in HMOs in free-world medicine, but there are important differences. In an HMO the evaluator decides whether the HMO will *pay* for the procedure. If the requested procedure does not meet HMO criteria, the evaluator will deny the request. The procedure can still be done, but the patient and their physician will have to find an alternative method to pay for it. Also, the HMO evaluator does not offer opinions on whether the procedure is appropriate or what could or should be done instead.

Correctional medicine UM is different. Those of us doing these evaluations aren't being asked about payment; we're being asked for permission to do the procedure at all. We cannot simply deny the request like an HMO can. If we don't think the procedure should be done, we must say what should be done instead: the alternative treatment plan.

When done poorly the ATP can irritate the primary care practitioner and even create an adversarial relationship between the site practitioner and UM evaluator. When done well the ATP is a written conversation between two equal colleagues, and the process can improve patient care.

Like any other bit of writing, it is important at the outset to define your audience. The ATP should be written with three potential readers in mind. The first is the site practitioner who made the initial request. A bad ATP will leave the PCP feeling underappreciated, threatened, and disrespected: *I don't trust you, and you are stupid.* A good ATP will leave the PCP feeling like you're on the same team and you have their back: *You're doing great! Let me help you!*

The second potential reader of the ATP is the adversary, like a plaintiff's lawyer or an advocacy group. A bad ATP will indicate you're denying the patient reasonable and necessary medical services. A good ATP will show nothing was denied and will not imply any medical service is off-limits.

ATPs are also read by nurses, who have to transcribe and record them into official records. A good ATP will make their life easier. A bad ATP can result in many hours of needless, morale-crushing busy work.

In my experience it doesn't take much more time to write a good ATP instead of a crappy one. Most UM evaluators, however, have never been taught how to write an ATP. Here is how I write mine:

1. *Restate what's being requested.*

The first sentence of the ATP should briefly summarize the case and restate what is being requested.

- 56 yo male s/p colonoscopy done for guaiac-positive stool. Request is for a routine postprocedure FU with the gastroenterologist.
- 63 yo male with reported gross hematuria. Request is for CT of the abdomen.

2. *Support your ATP.*

The next section contains the evidence that supports your ATP. This evidence can be pertinent positives, like x-rays, labs, and previous visits. It can also be pertinent negatives, like incomplete exams or missing data. Finally, this paragraph can also include pertinent research that supports your ATP, such as a quote from UpToDate, RubiconMD, or InterQual.

- The colonoscopy was negative except for a single sigmoid polyp. The pathology report on the sigmoid polyp is not attached to the report.
- There is little clinical information accompanying the request. I do not know if the patient has other medical problems, findings on physical exam, what medications he is on, or what labs have been done. Review of published treatment algorithms for the diagnostic

workup of hematuria (Essential Evidence Plus, UpToDate) shows CT is not the first diagnostic procedure that should be considered in most cases of hematuria.

3. *The ATP should defer the request, not deny it.*

It is important to never (or rarely) use the word *denied*. Instead you should restate what was requested and then say it is *deferred* pending whatever you want done instead, such as *pending receipt of missing information*; *pending complete evaluation of the patient at the site*; or *pending evaluation in a case review conference*.

- Routine post-procedure FU with GI is deferred pending complete evaluation of the patient and colonoscopy findings at the site.
- Abdominal CT is deferred pending complete evaluation of the patient at the scene.

4. *Tell the primary care practitioner what you want them to do instead.*

The next sentence contains instructions to the site practitioner. This is the actual ATP and should be labeled as such. I also always date the ATP.

- 3/11/2019 ATP: The site practitioner should obtain the pathology report on the sigmoid polyps and call me to discuss the case. The timing of follow-up colonoscopy will depend on the biopsy results.
- 3/11/2019 ATP: The primary care practitioner should do a complete physical examination, appropriate labs, and then discuss the case with me as to the next appropriate diagnostic procedure (ultrasound, cystography, etc.).

5. *State that whatever was requested can be reconsidered later.*

I always add this last sentence as well, to reaffirm I'm not denying any medical care. The request from the first paragraph can be considered later if clinically appropriate or any time if medically necessary.

- Off-site GI visit can be considered thereafter, as clinically indicated—or at any time if appropriate.
- CT can be considered thereafter, if clinically appropriate, or any time if medically necessary.

6. *Contact the PCP to let them know their request was ATP'd.*

I don't think PCPs should find out from a UM nurse that their request was ATP'd. They will feel much better about the process if you contact them. This also opens a method of communicating about the case if they have more questions. This can be accomplished with a simple email:

- Hi, Dr. X! Before we send this patient off-site to see the gastroenterologist, we need the biopsy report. If the adenoma is low risk, you can deliver the good news to the patient and tell him when his next colonoscopy will be scheduled. You'll be seeing him in chronic care clinic in the meantime.

- Hi, Dr. Y! I am attaching an algorithm for workup of hematuria. As you can see, there are several things that should be done before we consider a CT. Will you please call me to discuss this case?

Putting it all together, here are the full ATPs:

- 56 yo male s/p colonoscopy done for guaiac-positive stool. Request is for a routine post-procedure FU with the gastroenterologist. The colonoscopy was negative except for a single sigmoid polyp. The pathology report on the sigmoid polyp is not attached to the report. 3/11/2019 ATP: Routine post-procedure FU with GI is deferred pending complete evaluation of the patient and colonoscopy findings at the site. The site practitioner should obtain the pathology report on the sigmoid polyps and call me to discuss the case. The timing of a follow-up colonoscopy will depend on the biopsy results. Off-site GI visit can be considered thereafter, as clinically indicated—or at any time if appropriate.

  - Email to PCP: Hi, Dr. X! Before we send this patient off-site to see the gastroenterologist, we need the biopsy report. If the adenoma is low risk, you can deliver the good news to the patient and tell him when his next colonoscopy will be scheduled. You'll be seeing him in chronic care clinic in the meantime.

- 63 yo male with reported gross hematuria. Request is for CT of the abdomen. There is little clinical information accompanying the request. I do not know if the patient has other medical problems, findings on physical exam, what medications he is on, or what labs have been done. Review of published treatment algorithms for the diagnostic work up of hematuria (Essential Evidence Plus, UpToDate) shows CT is not the first diagnostic procedure that should be considered in almost all cases of hematuria. 3/11/2019 ATP: Abdominal CT is deferred pending complete evaluation of the patient at the scene. The primary care practitioner should do a complete physical examination, appropriate labs, and then discuss the case with me as to the next appropriate diagnostic procedure (ultrasound, cystography, etc.). CT can be considered thereafter, if clinically appropriate, or any time if medically necessary.

- Email to PCP: Hi, Dr. Y! I am attaching an algorithm for workup of hematuria. As you can see, there are several things that should be done before we consider a CT. Will you please call me to discuss this case?

Two more examples (minus email):

- 53 yo s/p treatment for tongue cancer in remission. Request is for routine FU with ENT at six months from last visit. The patient has finished all his radiation sessions. ENT note from 7/17 states the patient is in remission and the six-month FU visit is prn. The consult request notes no new symptoms. 3/11/2019 ATP: ENT consultation deferred. Per last visit with ENT, further visits are to be prn. The site PCP should evaluate the patient at six months from the last visit and again at one year. Off-site visit with ENT can be considered thereafter, as needed—or any time if clinically necessary.
- 62 yo who had a liver ultrasound as part of hepatitis C staging. The ultrasound showed a hypoechogenic polyp or cyst at the neck of the gall bladder. The radiologist says a CT may be of value. There is no report the patient is symptomatic. I submitted the case to a RubiconMD radiologist, who thinks this is an incidental finding and repeat ultrasound in six months is a better methodology to follow this incidental finding. 3/11/2019 ATP: Abdominal CT is deferred. Per RubiconMD radiologist's recommendation, the site PCP should order a follow-up ultrasound at around six months. CT may be considered thereafter as clinically appropriate (or any time if necessary).

COMFORT ITEMS:
THE SPECIAL PROBLEM OF CORRECTIONAL MEDICINE

COMFORT ITEMS

Perhaps the strangest aspect of practicing medicine in a jail or prison is "comfort" requests. This is when a patient comes to the medical practitioner and asks for something like a second mattress, the right to wear their own shoes, a second pillow, a second blanket, etc. This, of course, never happens in an outside medical practice. When was the last time you heard of a patient asking for a prescription for a pillow? Yet such requests are extremely common in correctional medicine. You might think, *Well, just give them the second pillow—what harm can it cause?* But it is not that simple. Like every medical issue, there is a right way and a wrong way to handle these requests. To understand why, let's consider the most requested comfort item in a correctional medical clinic: a second mattress.

When patients are first booked into a jail, they are issued (among other things) a mattress to sleep on. Jail mattresses are thin and not very comfortable, especially when placed over a concrete or metal bed frame. Why are they so thin? I have been told the main reason is security: The thicker a mattress is, the easier it is to slice open and hide contraband inside. Conversely, the thinner a mattress is, the easier it is for security personnel to find hidden contraband. While this may be true, I suspect a more important reason jails use thin mattresses is that they're cheap. Also, many jail administrators are OK with the fact that the mattresses are uncomfortable since, after all, jails are supposed to be punitive places.

When patients come to me complaining that the mattresses are not comfortable, I understand and even sympathize. Many aspects of jail life suck, including the mattresses. So if a jail patient says, for example, that sleeping on the thin mattress aggravates his chronic back pain, I tend to believe him. So why not just authorize the second mattress as medically necessary? The answer lies in the first rule of correctional medicine: fairness. If I authorize a second mattress for one patient with back pain, then the principle of fairness says I must authorize a second mattress for every patient with back pain. Otherwise, I have treated the first patient with favoritism.

This is why scoring a second mattress or second pillow can be a source of considerable prestige in jails and prisons. And not just prestige but money: Comfort items have value in the jail's black market. I learned this lesson the hard way early in my jail career when I authorized a second pillow for a patient and later learned this patient had been selling use of the pillow overnight to other patients in exchange for commissary items. Comfort items are valuable commodities.

Patients know all of this and expect me to be fair. That is why, if I authorize a second mattress for one patient, I will quickly get several more requests from others for second mattresses. "I also have back pain! I want a second mattress too!" And if I say no to these patients, many of them will file formal grievances. And rightly so! On what basis do I give a second mattress to one patient with back pain but not others? It is wrong to show favoritism.

But aren't there some patients with a legitimate medical need for a special mattress? Yes, there are! There is also a true medical device designed for those with a medical need for a special mattress: It is commonly called a hospital bed. I have had several patients in my career who needed to use a hospital bed while in jail. The most memorable was a patient who was quadriplegic and spent over a month in the county jail. Not only did we get him a hospital bed, but it was one of those high-tech beds that rotated slowly over time to prevent decubitus ulcers.

On the other hand, I can confidently say a double thin mattress is not a true medical device. It is not mentioned in any medical textbook I have ever found. A double mattress is, instead, a comfort item: It makes life in jail a bit more comfortable.

Some jails recognize this and have written objective guidelines as to which patients will be issued items designed to make jail life more comfortable, like a second mattress or second pillow. Examples are pregnant women after 20 weeks and those more than 70 years old. Some jail administrators make some comfort items, such as better-quality shoes and better food, rewards for patient workers or good behavior. Some jails put comfort items like extra pillows or shoe insoles on the patient commissary for purchase.

My personal opinion is that jail patients should have better living conditions than most do now, including better mattresses. And there is a role for jail medical staff to advocate for these changes. I believe this and have done so myself. However, the wrong way to do this is to medically authorize comfort items willy-nilly for some patients but not others.

The Best of Jail Medicine

Personal Shoes

Everyone who works in corrections is familiar with patients wanting medical authorization to wear their own shoes. A typical case would go something like this: "I have chronic back pain, and walking on these hard concrete floors makes it worse. Will you authorize me to wear my own shoes? You did last time I was in here, and it really helped."

We need to keep in mind, however, that allowing a patient to wear his own shoes gives that patient secondary gain. Shoes from home are, indeed, more comfortable than the typical jail sandals. Also, any patient who is granted a special privilege, like wearing their own comfy shoes, gains status among the other patients. When we approve inappropriate requests for "own shoes," we are bestowing prestige upon that patient. And we are denying that prestige to those whom we refuse. The unfairness of this is not lost on patients. Finally, "own shoes" are occasionally used to smuggle contraband into the facility. I remember one pair that had an ingenious hollow space carved out of the sole that was not easy to find on a typical security examination. If you routinely grant requests for "own shoes," you will inevitably get burned in this way.

The second important point is that it is the responsibility of the security staff to provide footwear to patients, not the medical staff. The question we are being asked in these encounters is this: Is there a *medical* need for this patient's own shoes? I've argued there is never a medical need for a second mattress. That is not the case for footwear.

Orthotics

There are indeed cases when special footwear is medically indicated. In fact, medically prescribed shoes have a medical name; they are called *orthotics*. Examples of orthotics are walking casts, splints like the CAM walker, and special shoes with, say, a special built-up heel for patients who have one short leg. The keys here are that orthotics are 1) prescribed by a physician and 2) fitted in a medical clinic. They are not purchased "off the rack" in a store. This includes arch supports patients can purchase in a store, like Dr. Scholl's.

So the first part of this quick and easy solution is this: Orthotics, as described above, may be approved on medical grounds for use within the facility. Orthotics must fulfill both criteria: They must be both prescribed by a physician and fitted to the specific patient in a medical clinic. It is not enough to just get your outside doctor to write you a prescription for your Air Jordans (as I have seen many times).

The second part of this quick and easy solution is this: The patient's own store-bought shoes are *never* medically indicated. This takes the whole issue of store-bought "own shoes" out of the medical arena entirely. There is no reason for a patient to go to the medical clinic to ask for them—it is not a medical issue. Such requests can be routed to security to handle. If they want to give "own shoes" to a patient, they may, but there is never a reason for a deputy to say to a patient, "The only way you will get to wear your own shoes is if medical approves it." In this system medical never does. In some jails security has taken over the shoes issue entirely. Medical is seldom involved.

However, there are a few special cases that require a special discussion.

What about diabetics and diabetic foot disease? Don't diabetics need special protective footwear?

In my mind this is debatable. Diabetics need to manage their diabetes properly and take care of their feet. I think they can do this wearing jail footwear. However, others disagree with me. The best solution I have found to satisfy both opinions is for the jail to purchase slip-on or Velcro sneakers, which medical can then prescribe to appropriate diabetic patients. Note that this makes them orthotics by definition: They are prescribed by medical and hopefully fitted in diabetic clinic, at which time foot care is reviewed as well.

What about patients with neuropathy of the feet?

The problem with nondiabetic neuropathy of the feet is that it is hard to objectively evaluate. Often it is what the patient says it is. I don't disbelieve my patient necessarily, but I also do not want to get into a situation where patients can get their own shoes just by saying their feet hurt and tingle. Once they figure that out, I will see a lot of patients with tingly feet. A better solution is to take patients with documented neuropathy (they have seen a neurologist, say, and had nerve conduction studies) and fit them with jail sneakers like the ones we discussed for diabetics.

What if the jail does not have the right-size shoes?

I call this the Shaquille O'Neal dilemma. What would you do if Shaquille O'Neal (7-foot-1 and 325 pounds) were booked into your jail? One immediate problem with Shaq is that he wears size 23 shoes. Your facility probably does not stock that size. (If your facility does, I'd like to hear about it!) In my mind this is not a medical issue, this is a clothing issue. If the facility does not have footwear this man can wear, one solution would be to allow him to wear his own shoes. However, this is not a medical issue. There is no need for a medical memo.

Are there any other patients who might qualify for more comfortable footwear?

There is a long list of other subjective complaints that could potentially be eased by more comfortable footwear. Rather than going into them one by one, a better solution is to place the jail sneakers we have already discussed in the commissary, where any patient can purchase them without having to go through the medical clinic. Outside of jail, if your shoes aren't comfortable enough, you don't go to a medical clinic. You go to a shoe store and buy better, more comfortable shoes. I think we should allow patients the same right by making jail sneakers available on commissary as part of the OTC commissary program. Consider making arch supports available as well. Some jails give these jail sneakers to the elderly and women in their third trimester of pregnancy as a comfort item.

Don't Do Doubles

A frequent complaint in jails comes from patients who request extra food for various reasons—they are underweight, they are just way hungry, whatever.

People who have been using methamphetamine in particular seem to arrive at jail ravenously hungry. At many facilities patients ask for "doubles," which means double food trays with every meal. "Doubles" are very popular with patients, as you might imagine.

In general, a request for extra food falls into the broad "comfort items" category that also includes requests for one's own shoes, double mattresses, extra blankets, warmer clothes, a bottom bunk, one's own bra ("Nothing at the jail fits!") etc. These requests are unique to correctional medicine. Nobody goes to a medical clinic outside of jail with the chief complaint of "I need a softer mattress" or "I need double portions at each meal, and my wife won't serve them to me."

The request for extra food is a little different from, say, a request for a double mattress because some patients really do have a legitimate medical reason for extra calories. Before we discuss such patients, however, there are several items that we should keep in mind.

1. Most correctional institutions offer between 2,500–3,000 calories per day to each patient. This is far more calories than the typical patient needs. A "quick and easy" calculation for the number of calories a person needs to eat to maintain their body weight is 12 times body weight (in pounds). For the standard 175-pound male (like me), that works out to 12 x 175 = 2,100 calories per day. If I were to eat a jail diet of 2,500–3,000 calories a day, I would gain weight. Because of

this excess of dietary calories, weight gain while in jail is a significant problem.

(As an aside, I remember seeing one patient who had just been released from jail waiting for his ride home wearing boxer shorts and carrying the pants he'd been booked in eight months previously—he could no longer fit into them. His boxer shorts had little hearts on them, no lie. Another patient gained so much weight he could no longer wear his dentures.)

The problem is even worse for women, who are generally smaller and need less food but who are served just as many calories as the men. A 2012 *Los Angeles Times* article, "Study Examines Diet, Exercise, Obesity in Prisons Worldwide," discussed this very problem.[1]

So even if underweight patients are not given access to extra calories, the standard correctional diet is usually enough for them to gain weight.

2. Most patients already have access to extra calories via commissary food. Of course, many patients do not have access to commissary, like those who are indigent and those with administrative sanctions (like lockdown). Also, there is at least a one-week wait in most jails from the time of booking until a patient can conceivably receive extra food items from commissary. The meth addicts arrive at the jail ravenously hungry and have a hard time waiting a week for extra food. Also, commissary food is mostly junk food with little nutritional value.

3. Patients often request extra food for nonmedical reasons. These include the ability to eat more of their favorite foods rather than foods they don't like, the ability to give extra food away as favors, and as a sign of increased status among other patients. Like it or not, extra food, whether it's "doubles" or diabetic snacks, is a highly desirable commodity in the patient economy. Those to whom we grant extra food gain privileged status and those whom we refuse resent it. This is an important principle, the principle of fairness. Ignore this one at your peril!

Using the Body Mass Index

Having said all this, the big question is, "Which patients would *medically* benefit from extra food?" The answer is patients who are malnourished. One objective sign of malnourishment is patients who are demonstrably underweight on a body mass index. A BMI of less than 18.5 is defined as underweight. A BMI of greater than 18.5 is defined as being normal weight.

Using 18.5 as a BMI cutoff makes it easy to identify patients who may benefit from extra calories. This can quickly and easily be done by the nursing staff. Patients who request "doubles" have their height and weight measured by the nurses and plotted on a BMI chart. Those with BMIs greater than 18.5 are told they are normal weight and do not qualify for extra calories. Those with BMIs below 18.5 have extra calories ordered and are scheduled for a recheck of their weight in one month. If their BMI then is over 18.5, the extra calorie order is rescinded. Patients with BMIs below 17 are deemed seriously underweight and scheduled into medical clinic for a complete physical to ascertain why they are so skinny. The nurses, of course, can refer anyone else to the medical clinic whom they are worried about.

At the Ada County Jail in Boise, Idaho, the nurses have placed a BMI chart next to the scale in the medical clinic waiting room along with an explanation of the 18.5 BMI cutoff. It is a common sight to see patients checking their BMI on the chart and then deciding not to submit a medical request.

'Doubles' Aren't the Best Way to Provide Extra Calories

For those patients who qualify for extra calories based on BMI, the next question is how to give them the extra calories. I believe authorizing "doubles" is a poor solution to this problem for several reasons:

1. "Doubles" double the calories you are serving the patient from 2,500–3,000 a day to 5,000–6,000 a day. That is a big jump! Most people cannot eat that many calories in one day even if they try. Most patients will do fine on, say, 1,000 extra calories a day.
2. A patient given two diet trays is not going to eat everything off the first tray and only then tuck into the second. Instead the patient is

going to eat the things he likes best off both trays (meat and potatoes, say) and not eat those things he does not like (like vegetables). In the interest of a healthy diet, we would prefer he eat his vegetables, but that is not going to happen.

3. Since the patient likely cannot eat everything on his two trays anyway, why not give extra food away to other patients as trade or for favors? The patient gets power and status from the extra tray, and lots of other patients will be jealous of this and want "doubles" too.

Instead of double trays, a much better way to provide extra calories is by giving qualifying patients 1–2 cans of supplemental nutritional drinks like Ensure or Boost each day—say, one at breakfast and one with dinner. I can tell you from experience that these have very little value in the patient economy. (You can prove this by putting them on the commissary and seeing how many you sell! They are not popular.) In fact, once you switch from "doubles" to Boost, your medical requests for extra calories will drop by 80%. No exaggeration.

There are other patients who will benefit by getting Ensure or Boost supplementation even though they might have normal BMIs. One example is alcoholics. Especially when they are going through withdrawal, they often have trouble eating. Often it is easier to get liquid calories into them (Boost) than solid calories. It is often the same story with chronically ill patients, like those receiving cancer chemotherapy.

Reference

1. Brown E. Study examines diet, exercise, obesity in prisons worldwide. *Los Angeles Times.* Published April 20, 2012. Accessed June 4, 2022. www.latimes.com/health/la-xpm-2012-apr-20-la-heb-prison-health-20120419-story.html

EYEGLASSES AND EYE EXAMS

Eyeglasses were partly why I got into correctional medicine in the first place. Sixteen years ago my local jail was under a federal consent decree and desperate to find someone willing to provide medical care to patients under its strict terms. They finally found me, reluctant as I was at the time. So for the first two years of my correctional medicine career, I operated under a consent decree that resulted from an ACLU lawsuit (may those days never return!).

One of the medical issues the ACLU was concerned about was patient eyeglasses. And so from the very beginning of my correctional medical career, vision complaints and requests for eyeglasses were a hot topic I had to deal with. In fact, I remember the very first medical clinic I did in the jail contained three or four patients wanting glasses. Since I am a slow learner, it took me several years to sort out in my mind how to deal with the whole issue. But I eventually figured out that vision complaints basically fall into four categories, and each should be dealt with in a different way.

1. *Distance vision*—Typical medical request: "I am having trouble seeing the television, and it is giving me headaches. I need glasses."
2. *Reading glasses*—"I am having trouble reading. I need glasses."
3. *Vision complaints with medical implications*—"My vision has suddenly gotten worse in my right eye."
4. *Routine screening exams*—"My yearly eye exam is overdue. Please schedule me to see the eye doctor."

Each of these requests should be handled differently by correctional facilities. If you set up a one-size-fits-all procedure for vision complaints, you will not be operating efficiently, and you will make mistakes. I would like to discuss each of these complaints in turn.

The Best of Jail Medicine

Distance Vision

There are four considerations when evaluating requests for distance-corrective lenses. The first is that the distant vista at which patients look is very different from the distant vista at which people outside jail look. On the outside there is a much greater need for distance-vision correction; after all, people who are driving need to clearly identify objects far away. *What is that object in the road a half mile ahead?* But what is the farthest vista to look at in one my jails? From one end of the pod to the other is, perhaps, 200 feet. When we say "distance vision" in corrections, we are talking about a totally different "distance" than outside jail. Instead of seeing things miles away, we are talking about seeing things within a room.

The second important consideration with glasses to help distance vision is whether there is a medical *need* for this type of correction. In fact, this is the only factor mentioned by the National Commission on Correctional Health Care (NCCHC) about glasses. Eyeglasses are defined by the NCCHC as "aids to impairment," which should be "supplied in a timely manner when the health of the patient would otherwise be adversely affected, as determined by the responsible physician."

But what does it mean that a patient's vision is so bad as to adversely affect their health? I interpret this to mean a patient's vision is so bad that they run into doors, for example. I have actually seen a few patients with vision this bad in my jails! It makes you wonder how they got along on the outside without glasses. For most other there is no medical necessity for distance-vision prescriptions. Wanting to see the TV better is not a medical issue by the NCCHC definition (in my opinion); nor is the complaint of "squinting at the TV gives me a headache."

The third factor to remember for any complaint of distance-vision problems is that glasses are not the only solution. If you are having trouble seeing a distant object, whether it is right across the room or a mile away on the next ridge, there are three ways to improve your ability to see that object. The first is with magnifying lenses. The deer hunter uses binoculars; the person in the room can put on glasses. The second is simply to *get closer.* The closer you get, the better you can see the object. The third way is to illuminate the object with more light. If you are having trouble reading a book in a dim room, turn up the lights.

All three methods work well. So if a patient complains they can't see the TV well, one legitimate piece of advice is simply to sit closer to the TV.

The final consideration for distance-vision correction is this: While there may not be a *medical* need for it, there may be an *institutional* reason a patient should receive distance correction. One example is the patient who is taking classes like the GED while incarcerated and needs distance lenses to see the instructor and whiteboard. You can move the patient closer to the whiteboard, you can increase the light on the whiteboard, and you can have the teacher write bigger, but it may be easier to just get that patient distance lenses.

Reading Glasses

This one is much simpler than the distance-vision problem above. Reading glasses are, of course, also not *medically* necessary. However, again, they probably are *institutionally* necessary. It is hard to argue with a patient who says, "I can't participate in my own legal case because without glasses I can't read my case documents or do research." Based on this argument, I think correctional facilities are obligated to have some mechanism of providing reading glasses to patients. The best way I have found to do this is to put reading glasses on the patient commissary. Reading glasses are not expensive; patients who want them can buy them. If a patient is truly indigent and wants reading glasses, just give him a pair. It is less expensive in terms of time and effort to do this than to deal with the inevitable grievances, indignant defense attorneys, and, of course, the ACLU (I know!).

Sudden Deterioration

This complaint, of course, has nothing to do with wanting glasses for reading or TV. This is a true medical complaint. This patient should go to the medical clinic ASAP and quite possibly needs an urgent referral to an eye specialist. There are many examples of eye complaints that arise from a medical condition. Examples include the patient with sudden vision decrease in one eye (in one case of mine due to a retinal detachment), a diabetic who is having decreased vision as a complication of diabetes, or an elderly patient with vision disturbances and headaches as a result of glaucoma or temporal arteritis. Individuals at high risk for medical complications of the eye include the elderly, those with chronic debilitating diseases like diabetes, and those taking anticoagulants. Correctional medical staff should have a basic understanding of the important medical disorders of the eye.

Overdue Exam

The question here is, how often do you do screening eye exams on patients who have no specific eye complaints? There are two entirely different screening eye exams that can be performed. The first is a refractory exam, consisting of visual acuity (like reading a Snellen chart) and an evaluation of the eye using an autorefractor. The point of this evaluation is to prescribe corrective lenses. We'll call this the *refractory* exam.

The second type of routine screening is the *medical* eye exam, which, of course, checks for diseases of the eye. The medical eye exam consists of, among other things, tonometry to measure eyeball pressure and pupil dilatation to allow detailed evaluation of the retina. These two examinations can be done at the same time but often are not.

One problem with setting up a program for routine eye exams in corrections is that there is no clear-cut community standard for these exams. Different insurance policies authorize different exam periods. For example, really good health insurance will pay for a complete eye exam yearly for life. But many insurance policies have the eye exam as optional or omit it entirely. Idaho Medicaid used to pay for yearly eye exams, but that benefit was cut a couple of years ago. There is only one guideline I am aware of: The American Optometric Association (AOA) has written a guideline that says children younger than 18 should have a yearly refractory eye exam. From 18–40 the AOA recommends every two years. After age 40, due to age-related diseases of the eye, the AOA says yearly eye exams should recommence.

Putting this all together, it seems to make a difference whether your facility is a juvenile detention center, jail, or prison. In jails, whether juvenile or adult, no routine refractory eye exams need be ordered until the patient has been incarcerated for one year unless there is a medical reason for an earlier eye exam, such as diabetes, hypertension, or severely impaired vision. In prisons scheduled eye exams of patients younger than 40–50 every 2–3 years seems reasonable to me. Yearly eye exams of patients in this age group seem excessive (even the AOA does not recommend exams that often!).

The main problem of patients older than 40 is the loss of near vision (as I myself have learned). Keep those reading glasses available! Patients older than 40 with preexisting health conditions that can affect the eye should probably get yearly eye exams. Whether healthy patients in their 40s without complaints need a yearly exam seems debatable to me.

Since the incidence of serious eye pathology goes up with age, older patients should again receive yearly medical eye exams, even if they are healthy and without complaint. I do not know what the optimal age for this transition is, however. Forty? Fifty? Fifty-five? Sixty? Make your choice!

WITHDRAWAL

THOUGHTS ON ALCOHOL WITHDRAWAL

I had a lot to learn when I began practicing medicine in county jails. One of the most important lessons was how properly to assess and manage alcohol withdrawal. In my previous life as an ER physician, I had seen a few alcohol-withdrawal patients and even one or two cases of delirium tremens (DTs). I thought I knew what I was doing. Wrong! I was first unprepared for the sheer number of alcohol-withdrawal patients I would see as a correctional physician. Alcohol withdrawal in jails is simply very common.

But I was also unprepared because much of what I had been taught about alcohol withdrawal was inaccurate or misleading. Nothing teaches like experience! After many years of treating a lot of alcohol withdrawal, I have gained some insights.

The onset of delirium tremens doesn't always fit standard timelines taught in textbooks.

Tintinalli's Emergency Medicine: A Comprehensive Study Guide, for example, says that DTs occur 3–5 days after the last drink. While this may be true in most cases, it was not at all uncommon for my patients to manifest severe alcohol withdrawal much sooner than this and also much later.

My record for the earliest manifestation of alcoholic delirium was a patient who manifested true DTs within 12 hours after his last drink. This patient became a frequent flyer and would reliably become delirious within 12 hours of arrest—until we learned to treat him early and aggressively.

On the other end of the spectrum, I had a patient who developed DTs on their eighth day after admission to the jail. It was so late I almost missed the diagnosis.

Alcoholic hallucinosis has been rare in my patients.

As taught in the textbooks, alcoholic hallucinosis is a syndrome that begins around 12–24 hours after the last drink and can last for 1–2 days. These patients typically see bugs or animals in the room (think the proverbial pink elephants). Patients with alcoholic hallucinosis are reportedly not disoriented and have normal vital signs.

I have only seen one patient with alcoholic hallucinosis that I know of over my entire correctional career. It has been exceedingly uncommon. I believe there are two reasons for this. First, alcoholic hallucinosis is thought to be related to thiamine deficiency, and my patients are relatively well nourished as a group. Second, like in most jails, my alcohol-withdrawal patients are given lots of thiamine as soon as they're identified—and for several days afterward.

The hallucinations of delirium tremens are unique "immersion" hallucinations.

The hallucinations of the typical DT patient are different from those of alcoholic hallucinosis and, indeed, from any other kind of hallucinations. The hallucinations of the DT patient are like this: The patient thinks he is in some other physical location and interacts with that location. For example, a DT patient could be fiddling with the wall at the back of his cell, and when you ask what he's doing, he will say, "I'm just trying to get this microwave to work." In his mind he is at home in his kitchen. Or he might be continuously trying to open the door of his cell, but in his delirium he's at the store and just trying to get its door open. DT patients are immersed in another time and place and interacting with that environment.

There is an intermediate stage of alcohol withdrawal not mentioned in textbooks.

Medical references like *Tintinalli's* and UpToDate typically divide alcohol withdrawal into two basic stages: mild and severe (or DTs). However, in my experience a recognizable syndrome of intermediate symptoms almost always precedes DTs: not eating, not sleeping, not stopping (relentless pacing), and tachycardia. This also means that once a patient has progressed to DTs, he usually is significantly dehydrated because he has not been eating. More important, if we can catch patients in this stage of withdrawal and recognize it as the "pre-DT syndrome," we can treat them more aggressively and perhaps avert delirium.

It takes exponentially more Valium to treat withdrawal the more it progresses.

I use Valium in my jails to treat alcohol withdrawal. You may use Librium or Ativan, and that is just fine. They all work.

Many patients can be successfully treated with a single 10-mg dose of Valium given early. If treatment is delayed until the patient has progressed and is sicker, it will take quite a bit more. But by the time a patient progresses to the stage of delirium tremens, he will need literally hundreds of milligrams of Valium—which is one reason why most cases of DTs should be treated in a hospital setting. Because of this, it makes sense to be liberal with Valium. One 10-mg Valium given early in the course of withdrawal can prevent the need for much, much more Valium later on.

Seizures due to alcohol withdrawal are a wild card—they can happen to anyone at any stage.

In my patients it is *not* true that those with more severe symptoms of alcohol withdrawal are at higher risk of seizures. In my experience patients with mild symptoms are just as likely to have seizures as those with more severe symptoms. Instead of the severity of withdrawal, the two factors that seem to correlate to the risk of alcohol-withdrawal seizures are:

Patients who have had alcohol-withdrawal seizures in the past are much more likely to have them again.

Patients who have been given Valium for alcohol withdrawal, even a single dose, are less likely to have a seizure.

In my cohort of patients, most who had alcohol-withdrawal seizures had not yet received Valium. In my mind this underscores the importance of treating alcohol withdrawal early.

CIWA-Ar has a couple of serious shortcomings (and many lesser ones).

The Clinical Institute Withdrawal Assessment of Alcohol Scale, Revised (CIWA-Ar) is the standard accepted way of assessing alcohol withdrawal used almost universally. CIWA-Ar scores the severity of the withdrawal state by assessing several symptoms. It also recommends treatment based on the patient's score. CIWA-Ar has been around since the mid-1990s and works OKish.

However, in my opinion, CIWA-Ar is a flawed instrument. It has at least two major problems and several minor ones. The first major problem is that it does not incorporate the single best objective measure of the severity of alcohol withdrawal: the heart rate. In my experience the heart rate corresponds very well to the progression of alcohol withdrawal. Patients with minor withdrawal tend to have normal heart rates—less than 100. As the severity of withdrawal symptoms worsens, so, predictably, does the heart rate. DT patients have markedly elevated heart rates—usually well over 150. I would be very concerned by a patient whose heart rate went up from, say, 80 to 110 even if her other subjective symptoms did not change. Heart rate is also an objective measure, as opposed to the CIWA-Ar scoring measures, which are all subjective.

The second major problem with CIWA-Ar is that it does not treat all cases of alcohol withdrawal. If a patient's symptoms are judged by CIWA-Ar to be too mild, CIWA-r says not to treat, despite the fact that the patient is, indeed, suffering from alcohol withdrawal. I have a serious objection to this. If we diagnose alcohol withdrawal, even in its earliest stages, we should treat it! Without treatment most of these patients are going to progress. With even a single dose of Valium, many will not. And what is the downside? There are times to be stingy with benzodiazepines— this is not one of them.

OPIOID WITHDRAWAL CAN BE DEADLY

One thing I always tell practitioners beginning jail medical practices: You're going to see a lot of withdrawal cases—study up! In particular, since the opioid epidemic hit, the number of patients I've seen in my jails withdrawing from heroin and other opioids has skyrocketed. I've seen enough patients withdrawing from opioids that I think I'm reasonably knowledgeable on the topic. Because of this I was quite surprised when I ran across this sentence in The Medical Letter:

Opioid withdrawal is not life-threatening.[1]

Although this sentence seems quite self-assured, it is flat-out wrong. In fact, it is not just wrong; it is also dangerous. People do die from opioid withdrawal. I know of several such cases from my work with jails. Opioid withdrawal needs to be recognized as a potentially life-threatening condition, just like alcohol withdrawal and benzodiazepine withdrawal.

There is no footnote to The Medical Letter's claim that opioid withdrawal is not life-threatening. Evidently this statement is thought to be "common knowledge." And, to be fair, I was taught this myself when I was going through my emergency medicine training in the 1980s. I suspect it was wrong back then as well as now. But it is also true that opioid abuse and withdrawal is different now than it was then.

Think about it: Nobody would dispute that patients withdrawing from heroin can get very sick. Some become seriously dehydrated from vomiting and diarrhea. Some get hyperdynamic, including tachycardia and fever. Between the two some develop significant metabolic acidosis. Anyone who has seen full-blown heroin withdrawal will tell you many of these patients look like crap. Opioid withdrawal can be a serious physiological stressor.

When heroin addicts are young and otherwise healthy, it is probably true that most can weather the storm of withdrawal. But in fact, not all heroin addicts in the modern era are young. I've seen heroin users in their 50s and 60s. And not all of them are healthy, even the young ones. Are you going to tell me opioid withdrawal cannot be fatal in a 55-year-old addict who also has coronary artery disease and diabetes? Or even that a young but debilitated and malnourished patient cannot be pushed over the edge by a nasty bout of cold-turkey opioid withdrawal?

There is also less pure opioid abuse now than there was back in the day. Nowadays heroin users commonly abuse other drugs as well. Modern street heroin may be spiked with short-acting opioids like fentanyl, sufentanil, or carfentanil. Opioid users tell me they shoot up Dilaudid, Suboxone, or whatever else they can get in addition to heroin. Finally, opioid users commonly combine other drugs with their opioid of choice. A common one is Xanax (which can be injected, snorted, or just swallowed), but I've also had heroin users tell me about concomitant use of stuff like Ambien, Seroquel, and even ketamine.

The bottom line is that opioid withdrawal in the modern era is more complicated and dangerous than the old conventional wisdom would have you believe. Opioid withdrawal may be more than simple opioid withdrawal if the patient has also been using Ambien or carfentanil.

All this needs to be kept in mind by the wise and canny jail practitioner. It is poor medicine to say, "Well, heroin withdrawal is not life-threatening" and so do little—or nothing. Jail practitioners need to take as much care with detox from opioids as they do with alcohol withdrawal. In my opinion all symptomatic opioid-withdrawal patients should be treated— every single one.

One reason why many jail practitioners hesitate to treat opioid withdrawal is there are some significant legal hurdles to using methadone and Suboxone. However, the alpha blockers work well too, and there are no legal hurdles to their use. Lofexidine has been successfully used in Europe to treat opioid withdrawal for many years and was approved in 2018 by the FDA for use in the U.S.[2] Lofexidine's cousin, clonidine, also works very well to mitigate the symptoms of opioid withdrawal, and clonidine has been around forever. In fact, a 2003 Cochrane review said, "We detected no significant difference in efficacy between treatment regimens based on clonidine or lofexidine and those based on reducing doses of methadone over a period of around 10 days"[3]

The "best" treatment for opioid withdrawal is a big subject for consideration on another day. My point here is that if you are unwilling or unable to use methadone or Suboxone in your jail to treat your opioid-withdrawal patients, then consider lofexidine or clonidine. Don't assume opioid withdrawal is not life-threatening and do nothing! Cold-turkey withdrawal is both cruel and potentially life-threatening.

Reference

1. Management of Opioid Withdrawal Symptoms. The Medical Letter. 2018; Issue 1554. Published August 27, 2018. https://secure.medicalletter.org/article-share?a=1554a&p

2. Basen R. FDA Approves First Non-Opioid Drug to Treat Withdrawal Sx. Medpage Today. Published May 17, 2018. www.medpagetoday.com/painmanagement/opioids/72938

3. Gowing L, Farrell M, Ali R, White J. Alpha$_2$ adrenergic agonists for the management of opioid withdrawal. *Cochrane Database Syst Rev.* 2003; 2: CD002024. doi: 10.1002/14651858.CD002024

HEROIN WITHDRAWAL

Imagine this: You're practicing medicine, and a patient comes to you with an illness. You make the diagnosis and say to the patient, "I can see you're very sick. There is a highly effective treatment for your condition that would make you feel a lot better. It's simple, and it isn't even expensive. But you know what? I'm not going to give it to you! You're not sick enough. Come back tomorrow. If you're sicker tomorrow—well, if you're *sick enough*—I will treat you then. But not right now."

Crazy, right? We'd never do such a thing.

But the problem is, we frequently do that exact thing with our heroin-withdrawal patients. I'm not singling out correctional medicine practitioners here. I think in general heroin withdrawal is treated better in correctional settings than it is in the community. Nevertheless, it is a fact that heroin withdrawal is often not properly treated in jails and prisons. I have seen it.

I believe there are four main reasons some facilities do not appropriately treat heroin (and other opioid) withdrawal.

1.   *They mistakenly believe cold-turkey withdrawal isn't dangerous.*

I was taught in my residency "no one dies from opiate withdrawal." This is a common belief to this day. The problem is that this is simply not true.

No one disputes patients can get very sick when going through heroin withdrawal. And maybe young and healthy patients can tolerate being that sick with no lasting problems. But what about someone who isn't that healthy to begin with? Say, someone who has asthma and heart disease? Or maybe an underlying sepsis acquired from sharing needles? What if this patient is also malnourished and dehydrated from not eating? Could such a person, already weakened by these conditions, end up dying when the physiological stress of withdrawal is piled on? Of course they could!

And they do. I personally know of cases where patients died while going through opiate withdrawal. But even if they don't, people get very sick from heroin withdrawal. To assume opiate withdrawal is a benign condition is a serious fallacy.

2.   *Clonidine is an effective treatment for heroin withdrawal.*

The second reason opioid withdrawal is often not treated is the mistaken belief that the only effective treatment is more opioids. And jail practitioners are reluctant to prescribe opioids for opioid withdrawal for various reasons. I understand this.

But the belief that the only effective treatment for opioid withdrawal is more opioids is also a myth. There is indeed a highly effective non-narcotic treatment for opioid withdrawal: clonidine.

I am talking here about using clonidine as a short-term treatment for acute heroin withdrawal in a correctional facility. I am not talking about treating the underlying opioid addiction itself. The treatment of opioid addiction commonly uses long-term prescriptions of Suboxone or methadone, known as *Medication for Opioid Use Disorder (MOUD)*.

I am a big fan of addiction MOUD, but treating withdrawal is different than treating addiction. When heroin users are booked into, say, a tiny rural jail for only a few days, it is sometimes simply not logistically possible to get them enrolled in a MOUD program. These patients are going to experience withdrawal. Let's treat that first—using clonidine.

Clonidine has been validated as an effective treatment for opioid withdrawal in several studies. I also have experience successfully treating literally hundreds of patients for opioid withdrawal with clonidine. I can tell you from long experience, it works, and it works well.

I understand the reluctance to use opioids in a correctional facility for heroin withdrawal, but I do not understand any reluctance to use clonidine, especially since clonidine is now in common use as a treatment for all sorts of other conditions, such as PTSD and nightmares.

3. *Don't use Benadryl to treat heroin withdrawal.*

The third reason heroin-withdrawal patients are not treated adequately for withdrawal is that some facilities use ineffective treatments such as diphenhydramine (Benadryl) or hydroxyzine (Vistaril).

Let me be simple and clear: Hydroxyzine is not by itself an effective treatment for heroin withdrawal! There is no medical literature to support using hydroxyzine in this role.

And why would anyone prefer Benadryl over an effective medication like clonidine anyway? One works, one doesn't. Benadryl is at best an adjunctive therapy. If you want to add Benadryl to a clonidine regimen for heroin withdrawal, I have no objection to that. Just don't use Benadryl as the main therapeutic agent.

A word about diarrhea: During heroin withdrawal patients commonly have diarrhea and abdominal cramps. Many facilities treat this with loperamide. I also have no problem with the use of loperamide as an adjunctive therapy to clonidine, but since the cause of the diarrhea is withdrawal, a more effective treatment for the diarrhea would be to simply give more clonidine. Clonidine treats the underlying cause of the diarrhea.

4. *COWS undertreats withdrawal.*

The final reason heroin withdrawal is often not adequately treated is reliance on withdrawal scoring systems that require patients to meet a certain minimum symptom score before they qualify for treatment. A protocol found in UpToDate using the Clinical Opiate Withdrawal Scale (COWS), for example, does not begin treatment until a patient has a COWS score of at least 8. That means a particular heroin-withdrawal patient could present with anxiety, muscle aches, chills, and nausea—and not get treated! We're back to "Come back tomorrow, and if you're sick enough, I'll treat you then!"

I suspect scoring systems like this are modeled after the alcohol-withdrawal scoring system CIWA-Ar, which also requires patients to hit a minimum criterion of sickness before starting treatment.

Personally, if a patient in one of my jails says he's a heroin user and starting to feel sick, I will start that patient on clonidine. I don't see the point of waiting. The clonidine will predictably make him feel better. And he'll be reassessed later to see if the dose is adequate or he needs more.

Benzodiazepine Withdrawal

Patients are dying in correctional facilities from benzodiazepine withdrawal. This is not just a theoretical observation—it really happens. This fact bothers me since benzo-withdrawal deaths are preventable. Benzodiazepine withdrawal is easy to treat! It is certainly easier to treat than the other two potentially deadly withdrawal states, alcohol and opioids. By far the most common cause of benzodiazepine deaths is, of course, not treating patients in benzo withdrawal!

Is your facility at risk of having patients die of benzodiazepine withdrawal? To find out, compare your policies to the following rules for the treatment of benzodiazepine withdrawal.

Treat everybody at risk of going through benzo withdrawal.

This includes *everybody* who has been taking benzodiazepines steadily for more than a month. It is usually not a problem to know who these patients are. You can call pharmacies and prescriber offices for details. Easier still, in most states you can check prescriptions of benzodiazepines (and other controlled substances) online using the PMP AWARxE database at https://bamboohealth.com/solutions/pmp-awarxe. Be aware, though, that patients can also get benzos illicitly online. Some also buy their benzos on the street. Be thorough in your evaluation of benzo use.

Don't use urine drug screens to exclude people from treatment.

Urine drug screens will not detect many benzodiazepines. Just because a patient's urine drug screen is negative for benzos doesn't mean they won't experience benzo withdrawal.

Don't use symptom scoring to exclude patients from treatment. And don't use CIWA-Ar at all.

It is true that patients going through benzodiazepine withdrawal can manifest many symptoms, including tremors, anxiety, psychosis, and seizures. However, it is possible for some patients to have minimal symptoms before they have a big event, like a seizure. Because of this you really should treat everyone at risk, even if they are not having symptoms. CIWA-Ar does not work for benzodiazepine withdrawal.

Know the big three predictors of a potentially serious withdrawal syndrome.

• Sudden cessation of benzodiazepine use

• Xanax (alprazolam) use

• High benzodiazepine doses

You must use a benzodiazepine to treat benzodiazepine withdrawal—period.

Some practitioners are so paranoid about the possibility of diversion and abuse of controlled substances inside their facility that they use other drugs to treat benzo withdrawal, like Benadryl (diphenhydramine). Don't do this. Benadryl does not work! There are times to be sparing in the use of controlled substances, but this is not one of them. You simply must use benzos to appropriately and effectively treat benzo withdrawal.

Don't use alprazolam (Xanax) to treat benzo withdrawal. Use a long-acting benzo instead.

By far the most prescribed and abused benzodiazepine is Xanax (alprazolam). Xanax has a short half-life, which tends to enhance its euphoric rush. This increases the danger of dependence for long-term users but also makes Xanax a poor choice to treat benzo withdrawal. If a patient needs to be withdrawn from Xanax, a far better and safer alternative is to substitute a long-acting benzo. I personally use Valium (diazepam), but Ativan (lorazepam) and Klonopin (clonazepam) are good alternatives. Begin by determining the equivalent doses of the long-acting agent and the Xanax using a conversion chart.

Taper slowly.

There is little evidence on the optimal duration or rate of tapering. In the absence of strong evidence, you can set up your own tapering schedule. I have seen several online. Most recommend starting at 50%–75% of the initial dose and reducing the dose by 12.5%–25% a week, with a longer taper the lower the dose gets. The higher the initial dose, the longer the taper will be (of course). A taper schedule of two months or more is not unusual, depending on the initial dose. It is also important to factor in other sedating medications your patient may be taking when coming up with an optimal schedule. Also (of course) monitor and adjust the taper as needed, depending on how your patient is doing.

Remember the first rule: *Treat everybody at risk for benzo withdrawal.* Treatment and tapering of any length are better than allowing an at-risk patient to go cold turkey.

THE MOST COMMON MISTAKE IN TREATING WITHDRAWAL

What is the most common mistake made when treating withdrawal in a correctional facility?

Consider these two patients:

A jail patient booked yesterday is referred to medical because of a history of drinking. He has a mild hand tremor and the look of a heavy drinker. But he says he feels fine and has no complaints. His blood pressure is 158/96, and his heart rate is 94.

A newly booked jail patient says she is going to go through heroin withdrawal. She is nauseated but still eating and has no gooseflesh or rhinorrhea. Her heart rate is mildly elevated.

In many jails neither of these patients would be started on treatment for withdrawal on their first visit to medical. But this would be a mistake! Both patients should be started on treatment for withdrawal immediately.

The most common mistake made when treating withdrawal in a jail is *not to treat the withdrawal at all!*

Both these patients have the potential to slide downhill rapidly. And in both cases the potential benefits of starting treatment far, far outweigh any potential liability.

Let's look at these cases in more detail.

Case No. 1

With this patient's history of drinking and look of a heavy drinker, he has a high risk of going through significant withdrawal. His hand tremor is already at least one sign. The problem is that the scale most commonly used to assess the severity of alcohol withdrawal, CIWA-Ar, would only score this patient as, at most, a 2 and does not recommend treatment for scores less than 8–10.

However, as we've discussed, CIWA-Ar is almost entirely subjective and relies heavily on patient cooperation in answering questions about symptoms truthfully and accurately. Many patients just don't provide accurate information. Maybe this patient is not a complainer. Maybe he is just cranky. Maybe he has some dementia. In the end there is a good chance CIWA-Ar has underscored this particular patient.

But even if CIWA-Ar has scored his current status correctly, what are his chances of getting worse over time? By not treating him you're gambling he will not get worse. I think if you look at the potential outcomes, that gamble is foolish. What do you gain if you are right, and he does OK over time? You saved one dose of Valium. On the other hand, what could happen if he has an alcohol-withdrawal seizure or otherwise deteriorates rapidly into serious withdrawal? He could suffer permanent harm. You will have to spend much more time and effort monitoring and treating him than if you had just treated him in the first place. You will have placed yourself at risk medicolegally.

In the end this patient should receive his first dose of Valium (or other benzodiazepine) now. There is no good reason to wait.

Case No. 2

Like the last patient, this woman is starting to show signs of withdrawal (tachycardia, nausea) and will assuredly get worse over time. Yet she also may not get treated immediately in the average jail. The temptation to not treat her heroin withdrawal comes from two sources.

First, many have the erroneous belief that opioid withdrawal does not kill patients the way alcohol withdrawal does, and therefore, cold-turkey withdrawal is OK. This of course is wrong.

Second, many believe methadone and buprenorphine (used in medication-assisted treatment, or MAT) are the only two drugs effective in treating opioid withdrawal. And since these two drugs are highly regulated and a hassle to prescribe and use, they are only used if a withdrawal patient gets sick enough. They are usually not given to every patient with mild opioid withdrawal.

However, the belief that only MAT works to treat opioid withdrawal is also incorrect. The alpha-adrenergic drugs clonidine and lofexidine work just as well as methadone in treating initial symptoms. Clonidine is not a scheduled drug, is easy to administer, and, if given in the correct dosage, is very effective in making heroin withdrawal more tolerable for the patient.

Patient No. 2 should immediately be given her first of several doses of clonidine and scheduled for routine reevaluations to see if she needs even more. Giving her clonidine now does not, of course, mean buprenorphine cannot be used later. But it does mean there again is no reason to deny treatment for this patient in early heroin withdrawal.

The most common mistake made in the treatment of withdrawal in jails is not to treat it at all. Don't make this mistake! Best medical practice is to treat everyone showing symptoms of alcohol or opioid withdrawal.

MEDICAL CARE

BEWARE THE BOUNCE-BACK

I learned about bounce-backs back in my emergency medicine days. A bounce-back is a patient you saw in the ER and discharged but who then returns within 48 hours with the same complaint. A lot of time is spent in emergency medicine education talking about how to handle bounce-backs. The basic message is, "Beware! You may have missed an important diagnosis the first time!"

Bounce-backs happen in correctional medicine too. They can happen in jails, where we often deal with patients we do not know well. But bounce-backs also happen in prisons when patients we know well have new complaints. Just like in emergency medicine, a bounce-back in a jail or a prison is a patient who comes to the medical clinic with a new complaint, receives a diagnosis and treatment, and then rekites for the same complaint within a couple of days. Here are a couple of examples.

- A jail patient comes to the clinic with a rash and is given a steroid cream for eczema. He returns in a couple of days saying the rash is worse and spreading.
- A prison patient complains of a cough and shortness of breath, is treated with an albuterol inhaler, and returns two days later saying his symptoms are worse.
- A patient returns with the same complaint of dizziness that you treated with antihistamines three days ago.

Clinicians who see the same patient for the same complaint may naturally feel irritation and frustration. I have myself! You think, *I just saw you for this! Give the treatment time to work!* There can be a tendency to feel threatened and even "double down" on the original diagnosis: "I know what I'm doing!" And most of the time, you will indeed have been correct the first time you saw the patient.

However, if you see enough bounce-backs, you will eventually find a patient in whom you missed an important diagnosis.

It is very important to remember this! In fact, we need to train ourselves to be grateful to such patients for giving us the opportunity to recheck our facts and conclusions. Such patients can save us from medicolegal disaster.

The following are general rules for dealing with bounce-backs.

1. Always do a more comprehensive physical exam the second time around. For example, on the dizzy patient, you could do neurological tests you may not have done the first time, like finger to nose, heel-to-toe gait, and rapid alternating movements. You could spend a little extra time looking for visual nystagmus. For the shortness-of-breath patient, you could listen long and hard to the heart and lung sounds and check for JVD and edema. Whatever you did the first time, when the patient bounces back, do a more thorough exam.

2. Seriously consider doing some other diagnostic test. This could be a lab, like a CBC and a chemistry panel or x-ray. A chest x-ray might be an excellent extra test for the guy who bounced back with shortness of breath.

3. Consider getting a second opinion from someone else, even if it's a "curbside consult" from a friend or an online service that offers medical advice, such as RubiconMD. This might be just the thing for the rash. I often take pictures of bounce-back rashes and send them to a friend who's a dermatologist.

After doing a more detailed exam and maybe something else, most of the time you will be left with the same diagnosis as before. If that is the case, you also should spend extra time explaining the diagnosis to your patient.

One cause of bounce-backs is patients who expect to get better sooner than they will. An example is the patient who sprained his ankle and bounces back in three days saying, "It's no better!" After doing an extrathorough exam and maybe ordering an x-ray, I need to explain to the patient that sprains typically take several weeks to heal. If I had done this the first time, perhaps the patient would not have bounced back!

What if a patient bounces back a second time? Again, do an especially thorough exam and then try something you did not before. This could be another imaging study or more labs. You could biopsy the rash. When patients bounce back multiple times, you should seriously consider getting a formal second opinion. This could be as simple as having a colleague see the patient or a visit with a specialist or even sending the patient to the ER.

Bounce-backs are an inevitable part of correctional medical practice. Take care to develop good habits with them!

Medical Refusal or Manipulation

A friend once asked about balancing the autonomy of patient decision-making and the risk to the facility of not providing appropriate care. He provided some examples:

1. An individual is on disability but wants to sign a waiver of responsibility so they can work.
2. A diabetic (NIDDM) individual wants to refuse their diet and be placed on insulin so they can eat whatever they wish.
3. An individual with a comminuted jaw fracture (wires were cut during an episode of nausea) now wants regular food despite oral surgeon advising limited jaw movement.

Writes my friend, "Documentation of appropriate examination and advice to the individual is, of course, the foundation of addressing the issue—but do you allow the 100% (physically) disabled person work; allow the diabetic to sign a refusal of the diet and prescribe insulin; give the individual with the broken jaw (who is asking for more hydrocodone) a regular diet?"

The issue is indeed a thorny one—when a patient wants to refuse strongly recommended medical care. Sometimes these are true refusals, meaning the patient understands the medical intervention being offered and truly does not want it. More often, though, such refusals are a form of manipulation to get something else the patient wants. I would like to address these two scenarios first and then discuss my correspondent's three specific examples.

Jail patients have the right to refuse medical care—even important medical care.

Medical Care   123

When people go to jail/prison, they lose the ability to make many everyday decisions. They no longer can wear anything they like; they have to wear jail togs. They no longer can eat whatever they like; they have to eat the food the jail serves (plus a limited commissary). What they can read, whom they can see and when—all these decisions are made by someone else. It's almost as if jail patients have regressed into being children again. It is tempting to think they have lost all their rights to choose, and that we, like parents of small children, can overrule any of their medical decisions we think are bad. This is a serious mistake.

And it is not true, of course. Incarcerated people do not lose their right to make their own medical decisions. They may decide to come to dental clinic—or not. If the dentist wants to pull a tooth, they may say no. They may decide to take their prescribed medications—or not.

However, refusing proffered medical care is not as simple as just saying no. For a refusal of medical care to be valid, four conditions must be met, whether the patient is in prison or a community clinic:

1. *Capacity*—Does the patient have the mental capacity to understand what's going on?
2. *Informed*—Has the patient been fully informed of the possible consequences of his refusal? Does he understand?
3. *Reversibility*—Refusals of care are not forever things. Patients may change their mind at any time.
4. *Documentation*—Each of these points must be appropriately documented, as well as the reason the patient gives for the refusal.

Let's consider each of these in more detail.

Capacity—Does the patient have the mental capacity to understand what's going on?

Most of the time capacity for refusal is obvious. Our patients who refuse medical care are typically sober, functioning adults. They look us in the eye, have normal interactive conversations, and are clearly fully sentient.

Capacity is trickier when the patient is refusing medical care but is intoxicated, demented, psychotic, or otherwise partially incapacitated. In these cases the practitioner must make the best decision they can based on the degree of mental impairment and urgency and immediacy of the medical need. Sometimes we may act against the patient's wishes. Sometimes the courts must decide the issue, such as in psychiatric cases. And sometimes we just have to wait for the patient to sober up and ask again later, when we know they have capacity.

Patients who are unconscious clearly do not have the capacity to refuse medical care. However, medical practitioners can still give care to unconscious patients if the medical need is urgent and immediate. I don't need a signed consent form to defibrillate an unconscious patient! The consent is assumed if the need is urgent enough.

Informed—Has the patient been fully informed of the possible consequences of his refusal? Does he understand?

To be fully informed patients must be told of the possible harms of their refusal, but that is not all. Patients must also understand the expected benefits of the therapy, the potential harms of the therapy (like side effects), and what the alternatives are. This seems like a lot, but in actual practice it does not take that long.

Besides, this is a conversation we ought to have even when the patient isn't refusing, though we commonly don't.

As an example, let's take the case of one of my patients who refused to take any medication for his seizure disorder. His rationale was that he didn't like the side effects of the medications he'd taken in the past, and since he only had seizures once every six months or so, he would rather have an occasional seizure than put up with being sedated.

This patient needed to be told of the possible consequences of his refusal (falls, injury, airway compromise, etc.) and that there were newer seizure medications (like Keppra) with fewer side effects. If he still refused (and he did in this case), so be it. We documented the conversation and went to the next step.

Reversibility—Refusals of care are not forever things. Patients may change their mind at any time.

A common mistake made by healthcare providers when their patients refuse care is to treat the refusal as a permanent, unable-to-be-changed decision. Not true! And this is critically important. Patients have the right to change their minds. And in fact, we should want them to!

Besides being told about the possible consequences of any refusal of medical care, every patient should also be told they may change their mind at any time and to let us know if they do.

Besides this, there are many circumstances when healthcare providers should ask again about a medical refusal. For example, a patient may refuse medical care when they're drunk but be more rational when they sober up. I once had a renal patient who told me he would not allow any dialysis as long as he was in jail. "I don't care if I die," he said. But he was still intoxicated during this rant! By the next day he was sober and allowed us to take him to the dialysis center.

It's almost always a good idea to inquire about medical refusals after a period. How long this period should be depends on the urgency of the therapy. In the case of the dialysis patient, it was the next day. Many schizophrenic patients are ambivalent in their decision-making, so I may ask them if they will take their meds again in an hour. If a prison patient refuses statin therapy for his cardiovascular risk, I may not reask about the refusal until his yearly chronic care clinic visit.

Documentation—Each of these points must be appropriately documented, as well as the reason the patient gives for the refusal.

Probably the most common mistake made by medical providers when dealing with refusals is not documenting the encounter adequately. The documentation usually does not have to be very long. I usually document the reason the patient gives for refusing, plus one sentence for each of the three areas noted above:

Mr. Smith refuses to allow me to do an I&D of an abscess on his leg. He says he thinks he is going to get out of jail after court today and will have the abscess taken care of by his regular doctor. He understands the risks of refusing the procedure at this time. If he is not released, I will reevaluate the abscess tomorrow.

It took me 60 seconds to write that out (I timed it).

Sincere Refusal or Manipulation?

Of course, the cases my friend presented are not examples of sincere and rational refusals such as Mr. Smith's. In these cases the patients appear to be manipulating the system to get something they want. The critical difference in these cases is that the patients want my friend to give them something he does *not* think is legitimate medical therapy. They aren't refusing a treatment he's recommending; they are demanding a medical therapy he doesn't think is appropriate.

I have run across every one of the situations he wrote about. However, the most common type of this type of manipulation I run into is the request/demand for a medication I don't want to prescribe—such as gabapentin.

Dealing with attempts at verbal manipulation like this requires the skills of verbal jiujitsu. These are not intuitive to many medical practitioners.

However, the core insight in these three cases is that we do not have to give any patient medical therapy we think is inappropriate. I don't care that the first patient wants to revoke his disability status; if I don't think he's medically able to work, I'm not going to certify that he can. That's my decision, not his. I'm not going to allow a patient with a fractured jaw to ruin the surgical repair by having inappropriate food. Whether to prescribe insulin is my decision, not the patient's. And really, the decision to prescribe insulin is not based on whether patients will be compliant with their diet. I assume many of them won't. In fact, even if diabetic patients eat diabetic trays, I assume many will continue to eat crap from the commissary.

The second core principle of verbal jiujitsu relevant to these cases is that there is safety in numbers—the more medical practitioners agree on a decision, the stronger and safer the decision is. So if these were my cases, I would make sure the patients know I am not the sole decider.

The Three Cases

In the case of the broken jaw, I am not the one who ordered the soft diet—the oral surgeon did. So I would call the oral surgeon and tell him the patient's wires had to be cut due to nausea and the patient now wants a full diet. I suspect the surgeon will either reattach the wires or say "no way" to a full diet until he sees the patient (either way, problem solved).

In the case of the patient on disability who wants to work, the answer depends on who granted the disability status. If the patient has formal federal disability benefits and is receiving disability payments, of course I can't rescind that. If I, myself had previously placed this patient on an "unable to work" status and I truly believe he should not work, then I would treat this request like an appeal of that decision. As a response to the appeal, I would discuss the case with other people who know the patient and have a stake in the outcome, like other practitioners in the jail, the director of nursing, the health services administrator, and maybe even the jail commander. I suspect all would agree on the correct medical course of action. I would then tell the patient the decision (and document this, of course).

Finally, there is the case of the type 2 diabetic patient refusing a diabetic tray. That is his right. I assume many of my diabetic patients sabotage their diabetic diets anyway by eating commissary food. However, this patient mistakenly believes insulin will allow him to eat anything he wants and still be healthy. The issue here is that this patient has a serious misunderstanding of how type 2 diabetes works!

I had a similar patient in my jail who told me, "My (outside) doctor told me I could eat anything I wanted as long as I took my diabetic medication." This is so wrong as to almost be medical malpractice if the doctor (really a PA in this case) actually said it.

Insulin cannot compensate for diet in type 2 diabetics because they are all insulin-resistant. This means, of course, that insulin does not work perfectly well with them. The flip side of insulin resistance is that type 2 diabetics are carb-sensitive. Sugar and junk carbs will increase their blood sugar in an outsize way compared to nondiabetics. Since they are also insulin-resistant, insulin cannot fully compensate for this. The only real solution is to reduce the carb burden the insulin has to work on.

Because of this, the decision to start insulin in a type 2 diabetic should be based on the length of time they have had their disease and their A1C level, not on a vague promise to keep to their diet.

The real issue in this case is not the request for insulin but the refusal to adhere to a diabetic diet. This patient needs to know insulin is not a "cure" for diabetes and will not compensate for eating crap food. He also needs be informed that the possible consequences of eating junk carbs can be blindness, impotence, amputations, strokes, heart attacks, etc. He needs to know the best therapy for type 2 diabetes, by far, is to stop eating crap (and what crap is), exercise regularly, and lose a bunch of weight. This would be far more effective than insulin ever could be.

As we discussed, this conversation should be documented. And his refusal should not be considered a forever decision. The whole conversation on the importance of diet and consequences of refusing to eat right should be repeated and documented at every chronic care visit.

DOCUMENTING TEST RESULTS
THE ED AND MIDGE WAY

I have a senior Yorkie named Ed. Ed is experienced and knows the daily routine of our house. Last year we got a Yorkie puppy named Midge. She initially knew nothing. It has been entertaining to watch Ed educate Midge on what to do. Midge watches Ed closely and then does whatever Ed does. She is a true Ed Mini-Me. If Ed lies down, Midge lies down. If Ed asks to go out, Midge wants to go out too. If Ed begs for a treat, so does Midge.

Since Ed is a pretty good dog, most of what he has taught Midge has been positive, like to ask to go outside when you need to potty and sit to say "please" when you want a treat. But Ed also has some bad habits he has imparted to Midge. Ed still has the Yorkie propensity to yap at the door when the doorbell rings, and so Midge has also learned to sound the alarm.

Medical education is like this. I remember being a young-dog medical intern and watching my heroes, the senior residents. Not everything in medicine is taught in textbooks and didactic lectures! Much of what we actually learn as medical practitioners is an imitation of our elders. For example, I watched what the senior residents ate (junk), when they slept (rarely), and how they treated nurses (often poorly), among other things. Like Ed, most of what my senior residents taught me by example was good. But there are a few sketchy practices handed down from medical resident to medical student that can become bad habits.

One of these is how to document results of tests, like lab tests and x-rays. I can still see one of my old senior residents sitting at a desk back in the day with a large stack of lab tests. He would scan each of them for a millisecond and then scrawl his initials and the date at the bottom. This supposedly showed he had reviewed the lab results. But it really showed no such thing! Perhaps the resident also scrawled *WNL* to mean *within normal limits*. One old joke from my residency days was that *WNL* really meant *we never looked*!

Instead, the proper way to way to document test results is to interpret them! Interpreting test results doesn't take much more time that the old signature/date scrawl but conveys much more information. Interpreting test results consists of three parts.

First, state briefly why the test was ordered. Each test should have been ordered for a specific reason (otherwise, why did you order it?). This takes one sentence:

- *CBC and CMP done as part of yearly wellness exam.*
- *CXR done to check for pneumonia in a patient with fever and cough.*
- *Leg ultrasound done to look for DVT in a patient with swelling.*

Second, interpret the test in light of why it was ordered.
- *Pap smear shows resolution of previous LSIL.*
- *No active TB seen on CXR.*
- *Clean catch UA shows hematuria.*

Third, state what will be done about the test result. Will it change the patient's treatment plan?
- *No anemia found. No change in therapy needed.*
- *U/A shows pyuria. Will start antibiotics and FU in clinic one week.*
- *TSH low. Will decrease levothyroxine dose and recheck in three months.*

Finally, studies ordered for one reason sometimes come back with significant findings unrelated to that reason. I'm not talking about a CMP with a couple of values barely out of range; almost every lab panel will have a couple of mild abnormalities due to simple random fluctuations. I mean important unexpected findings that you also need to mention, interpret, and create a follow-up plan for. A good example would be a CXR done because of a positive PPD that is negative for active TB but shows an unexplained pulmonary nodule.

- *CXR done for positive PPD shows no active TB. There is a pulmonary nodule. The radiologist recommends chest CT, which I will order.*

So that is the process! It is not hard. Here are some complete examples:

A new patient at a jail says her last Pap smear was abnormal. Proper interpretation of the records when they arrive:

- *Old records ordered for last Pap results. This was done on 6/15/2020 and showed ASC-US. Will schedule FU Pap six months from last test (12/2020).*

An EKG is ordered because a patient is having chest pain to see if he is having acute ischemia. Proper note:

- *EKG done for atypical chest pain shows no evidence of acute ischemia. Will repeat in three hours.*
- *Metabolic panel ordered to assess renal function in a diabetic. BUN and creatinine show normal renal function. Will repeat in chronic care clinic one year. Incidental finding is markedly elevated liver enzymes. Hepatitis screen ordered.*
- *CBC ordered due to history of anemia. Results are normal. No treatment needed.*

This may seem like a lot, but it's really not. Once you get into the habit of documenting like this, it becomes second nature. This method works especially well in electronic medical records, where it is easy to type the study interpretation into a chart note or appendix to the original clinic note.

If we all get into the habit of documenting this way, the younger practitioners we train will naturally pick it up, just like Midge and Ed!

Patient Weight Is a Powerful Diagnostic Tool

Patient weight is a powerful diagnostic tool that is underutilized in corrections. The reason for this, probably, is that not much attention is paid to weights in outside medicine. In a general medical clinic, say, a patient's weight could be compared to their last routine visit, and some general conclusions might be reached, such as, "You've gained 10 pounds since last year. This is not good for your general health."

However, things are different in corrections. Our patients are with us all the time—they never go home. Many are "frequent flyers" in the medical clinic, either due to their medical problems or because they complain a lot. I have found patient weights in correctional clinics are a gold mine of useful information—so much so that I think a patient weight should be the fifth vital sign.

Let me give you several situations where weights will help you. Often the patient's weight is the only objective evidence you have to assess a complaint!

1. *"I've lost 30 pounds since I came to this jail and had to eat this stinking food."*

    I have heard this complaint a surprising number of times. If your facility weighed this patient at admission, you would know immediately if this claim was valid. When I have an admission weight, often I can reply, "Actually, your weight at booking was 178 pounds, and your weight now is 180 pounds. You have gained weight, not lost it."

    If you don't know what the patient weighed at admission, it's a hassle. All you can do is track the patient's weight from that point forward and document that there is no further significant weight loss. This, obviously, is more work than being able to say, "No, actually, you haven't lost a significant amount of weight."

2. *"I haven't kept anything down for the last three days."*

If you have a baseline weight to work with, it will help you decide how to approach this patient. Let's say this patient's baseline weight was 145 pounds, and her weight today in clinic is 146. In that case her claim of having kept nothing down is probably an exaggeration. On the other hand, let's say her weight today is 141. She may have lost several pounds. I would be much more likely to consider IV hydration in addition to antiemetics.

Either way I can use her weight to monitor her response to whatever therapy I use. If her weight is down and I aggressively hydrate her, I expect her weight to return to around 145 within a day or two. I do not want her to drop more pounds.

3. *"I'm constipated. I haven't had a bowel movement in six days."*

Again, a baseline weight can help you evaluate this complaint. Let's say his baseline weight was 166 pounds and his weight today is 165. A one-pound weight loss is not congruent with a claim of no bowel movement for six days.

4. *"I'm retaining water. Look how much my legs are swollen. I need a water pill."*

This complaint is worth a detailed discussion. Suffice it to say here that if this patient's weight is stable, her ankle swelling is likely due to dependent edema rather than water retention. The appropriate therapy is not diuretics; rather, she should be instructed to elevate her legs when she can, exercise, walk, and possibly use TED hose.

5. *Type 2 diabetics*

I have noticed that some type 2 diabetics lose weight in jail—sometimes a lot of weight, probably because they can't raid the refrigerator for Ben & Jerry's at 2 a.m. If you have a documented weight loss in a particular diabetic patient of, say, 50 pounds, you often can seriously step down their diabetes therapy.

The Best of Jail Medicine

6. *Hunger strikes*

If a patient eats nothing and does not exercise, he will lose approximately a pound a day. You can use serial weights to monitor this. If a patient is losing less weight than this, he is probably eating something. On the other hand, I had one patient who would hand back empty trays, indicating he had eaten. However, his weight kept dropping. It turned out that he was skillfully throwing away most of his food in the toilet.

Do you have other examples where weights helped you make a diagnosis? I would like to hear them!

An Approach to Chronic Pain

One of the most fearful and frustrating events in my correctional medicine world used to be when a new chronic pain patient would arrive in my clinic. A typical patient would be a Ralph, a middle-aged man who has had chronic back pain for many years. Ralph has had a couple of back surgeries, steroid injections, and more than one kind of stimulator, none of which has been effective. He arrived at the jail taking a long list of sedating medications such as muscle relaxers, gabapentin, and sleeping aids, plus, of course, big opioids. In addition Ralph has alcohol abuse issues. The reason he is in jail is a felony DUI charge. Now he is in my medical clinic, looking expectantly at me. How am I going to fix his pain problem?

The answer, of course, is that I am not. I am not that smart. He has already seen lots of doctors, including pain specialists and surgeons, who have tried almost everything that can be tried, and they have not fixed his chronic pain problem. I'm not going to be able to either. In my opinion the most common and serious mistake made in the treatment of chronic pain in corrections is when we imply that we can eliminate chronic pain.

It is an easy trap to fall into. It works like this: Ralph will say, "I have chronic pain. You are now my doctor. What are you going to do about my pain?" And I would reply something like, "Well, let's try *x*." *X* could be NSAIDs, gabapentin, duloxetine—anything, really. What Ralph understands, though, is that whatever I have prescribed should reduce or eliminate his pain. Why else would a doctor prescribe it?

But of course it does not eliminate Ralph's pain. How often has one of your chronic pain patients come back and said, "You did it, doc! After years of chronic pain, that meloxicam prescription finally did the trick!" None of mine have ever said that either.

No, inevitably, Ralph will say, "I'm still having pain." "Well, let's try *y*, then," I'll say. Of course, *y* won't eliminate his pain, either. Repeat this pattern a couple more times, and a severely dysfunctional dynamic has been firmly established. Since nothing I prescribe works, Ralph suspects I am not competent. A better doctor would have figured this out! Eventually, Ralph and other chronic pain patients become frustrated, angry, and distrustful. The clinical encounters become adversarial and unpleasant. We doctors dread seeing these patients.

But it does not have to be this way! The root problem here is that, without meaning to, I have set the wrong treatment goal for my patient—a treatment goal I cannot achieve. I cannot eliminate Ralph's chronic pain. I should not imply I can.

According to a great 2017 article published in the *Journal of the American Medical Association,* titled "Primary Care of Patients With Chronic Pain," I need to have a long conversation with Ralph in which I make clear that elimination of his pain is not likely to happen. Instead, he and I need to focus on his lifestyle and keeping him active.[1]

These authors say, "The primary goal of caring for the patient with chronic pain is not the elimination of pain but the improvement of function."

This simple sentence has totally transformed my approach to chronic pain patients. The result has been that we get much more accomplished, I don't dread seeing them, and they are happier. My chronic pain patients and I are no longer adversaries.

Now when I see chronic pain patients like Ralph, the first thing I do is come right out and say, "I am not going to be able to cure your chronic pain. No one can cure most cases of chronic pain. If I could cure chronic pain, I wouldn't be here—I'd be spending my millions of dollars on some beach in the Caribbean. [That usually gets a laugh.] To some degree, you're going to have to learn to live with your chronic pain. I will help you with this."

We will then discuss Ralph's level of activity. If he is the Most Valuable Player in the prison basketball league, I probably have little to offer him (don't laugh; this was an actual chronic pain patient). More likely we will set a goal of improving his activity level. If he is in a wheelchair, I want him using a walker. If he uses a walker, I want him to progress to a cane, and so on. For most of my chronic pain patients, I mainly want them not to vegetate in their cell. I want them walking in their dorm and in rec. I'll ask Ralph to track how much he walks and report back to me. I want him to increase his range of flexibility as well.

What I have asked Ralph to do is hard work, and he will need help. One of my jobs is to get him this help by asking my colleagues for their expertise. This is a *multidisciplinary approach* to chronic pain. For example, many (if not most) chronic pain patients have mood disorders, usually depression, because dealing with chronic pain can weigh one down. I'll arrange for Ralph to see a mental health professional. Ralph and most other chronic pain patients should also see a physical therapist, and so I'll arrange that, as well. Cognitive behavioral therapy (CBT) can be thought of as formal instruction on techniques for dealing with incessant chronic pain. CBT has been shown to improve function in chronic pain patients and is well worth the effort to set up at your institution.

I'll also use medications, but medications must be tied to increasing function. If I prescribe gabapentin, say, it will be tied to a specific objective goal, such as walking with a walker instead of using a wheelchair or flexibility I can easily measure in my clinic. If the objective goal is not met, the medication has failed and will be stopped.

One great advantage of this approach is that I can objectively measure how well Ralph is doing. By using function as a goal, I can verify whether Ralph has reached his goals. Notice also that I am no longer responsible for Ralph's pain. Instead, I am giving him resources to help him manage his own problem. The shift in responsibility here is huge! I can tell you this shift in approach to chronic pain has made me a much more effective physician to my chronic pain patients.

Reference

1. Schneiderhan J, Clauw D, Schwenk TL. Primary Care of Patients With Chronic Pain. *JAMA*. 2017; 317(23): 2367–68. doi:10.1001/jama.2017.5787

Food Allergies

In my previous incarnation as an emergency physician, I saw a lot of cases of acute allergic reactions. It is a very common emergency complaint; I have probably seen hundreds in my career. But when I began my jail medicine career, I was still unprepared for the sheer volume of food allergies claimed by patients. Who knew so many patients had so many food allergies?

Of course, most of them don't. Most just don't want to eat something on the jail menu. Patients believe that if they claim an allergy to a food they dislike, you cannot serve it to them. They will claim allergies to tomatoes, onions, mayonnaise, etc., when really they just don't like these foods. Tuna casserole doesn't seem very popular for some reason.

However, some patients truly are allergic to some foods, and we can potentially harm them by ignoring their complaints. How do correctional medical staff sort out the truly allergic from the "I don't like it" crowd? It is an important question because we certainly don't want anyone in our care to have a sudden anaphylactic reaction!

To answer this question, we need to understand the mechanism of food allergies; the overall incidence of food allergies, as well as their incidence of death; how to accurately diagnose a true food allergy; and what steps to take once we find one. All of this is important to make accurate risk assessments.

Understanding Food Allergies

The incidence and causes of food allergies vary markedly with age. For the most part food allergies are a problem of childhood. In children the most common food allergies are to milk, eggs, wheat, and nuts. However, most of these allergies abate with time. So a child who is allergic to eggs most likely will be able to eat eggs as an adult. One important exception to this rule is peanuts and tree nuts (like almonds, cashews, etc.). Those allergies tend to persist into adulthood. The most common adult food allergies are peanuts, tree nuts, shellfish, and fish.

True allergic reactions to foods come in two types. The first is called *IgE-mediated* allergic reactions because the IgE antibody is essential to the reaction. The second type does not involve IgE and so, of course, is called *non-IgE-mediated*. The best example of this is celiac disease, in which patients are allergic to gluten found in grains. Non-IgE-mediated allergic reactions are typically indolent and chronic and may not be discovered for several years.

IgE is an antibody created by the body to react to a specific antigen substance. This substance can be ragweed pollen, of course, but it also can be food proteins. Later on, if the person eats the same food that triggered the creation of IgE, the protein locks onto the IgE, causing the release of inflammatory chemicals such as histamine, cytokinins, prostaglandins, and leukotrienes.

The most common symptom caused by these inflammatory chemicals is hives, the itchy, splotchy rash we have all seen. The second most common is angioedema, which is swelling of the face. Angioedema most commonly occurs around the eyes but also rarely can cause the tongue to swell. Third and less frequently, the allergic reaction can cause bronchospasm in the lungs, so the patient wheezes as if having an asthma attack. Finally, the patient can suffer anaphylaxis, which consists of acute vasodilation leading to hypotension, shock, and possibly death.

All these allergic symptoms occur within minutes of eating. Allergic hives that occur several hours after eating are probably not due to the food.

Of these allergic symptoms by far the most common are hives and angioedema. However, most of the time hives and angioedema are nuisances rather than life-threatening emergencies. On the other hand, anaphylaxis is an acute medical emergency. Anaphylaxis is the allergic reaction we should fear the most and work to prevent.

The Centers for Disease Control and Prevention estimates that approximately 100 deaths from food allergies occur in the United States each year. Almost all the reported deaths occur in teenagers or young adults who knew they were allergic to the food they ate. By far the most common culprit foods are peanuts and tree nuts (85%), with shellfish coming in second. In contrast, 400 deaths due to allergic reactions to penicillin occur every year, and most of those occur in people who have no idea they are allergic.

Risk Assessment Tips

You can use these principles to do a risk assessment for individual patients. Patients at higher risk of an anaphylactic allergic reaction are those who are younger (late teens, early 20s) who state an allergy to peanuts, tree nuts, or shellfish and who have had a previous documented allergic reaction. Patients with a lower risk are older patients who state an allergy to a low-risk food (say, onions or peppers) and cannot document a previous severe allergic reaction. Someone who has had a severe allergic reaction to a food in the past should be able to tell you about an emergency room visit, allergy testing, EpiPen prescriptions, and how they avoid the food in restaurants and while shopping.

However, there are other tests that can help you sort out the confusing cases. The first is an IgE test. This is a blood test that measures the levels of IgE to a certain specific allergen—say, peanuts. A positive result would be a peanut-specific IgE of greater than 2.0 kU/L. If the test comes back at, say, 0.35 kU/L, then the patient is not allergic. The test is quite sensitive but not specific. That means you can believe a negative result, but patients with positive results might still not be allergic.

A second test is the skin prick test. The patient's skin is pricked with a small instrument, and a drop of allergen extract is placed on the site. If a patient is truly allergic, they will form an itchy wheal at the site within 5–15 minutes. The advantage of this test is that it is cheap and easy to do, and the results are immediate. If need be, you can send patients to an allergist for skin prick testing.

"Food challenge" tests probably should not be done in a correctional setting. This is where you simply feed the food to the patient and wait to see what happens. If this is done in a double-blinded fashion, it is the most accurate test of all. However, sometimes patients will have done their own food challenge without knowing it. For example, a patient might say they are allergic to eggs but admit to eating pasta and mayonnaise, both of which are made with eggs. They are likely not truly allergic.

Setting Policies

Of course, the easiest way to deal with the foods most likely to cause severe allergic reactions is not to serve them at all. Most jails do not serve shellfish to patients. (If your jail does, write to me; I would like to know about it!) If your facility uses tree nuts in cookies, consider eliminating them from the menu. Then you won't have to worry about it. That just leaves peanuts as the food served in most prisons and jails that has the greatest potential to cause allergic reactions.

Once you have discovered a patient has a positive IgE test to peanuts, what should you do? It may not be enough to simply order a peanut-free diet. Since allergic reactions can be triggered by even a small amount of allergen contact, you should consider these other factors:

1. You probably have peanut-containing items on your commissary. Should this patient have a commissary restriction?
2. Should this patient be allowed to work in the kitchen, preparing peanut butter sandwiches?
3. Should this patient be housed with other patients who may be eating peanut butter sandwiches right next to him?
4. What about an EpiPen? Where should it be kept?

I hope this information will make you a little more confident the next time a patient says they are allergic to, say, "all vegetables" (as a patient told me once). You can also use these principles of risk assessment, history, and testing to write a policy and procedure for the clinical assessment of food allergies.

The Best of Jail Medicine

BEHAVIOR

Manipulation

One of the more common complaints I hear from correctional practitioners (especially new ones) is, "Manipulative patients are driving me crazy!" To be honest, I ran into a lot of manipulative patients when I worked in the ER as well. ERs are the epicenter of narcotic drug-seeking! But it is true that many of our patients in corrections are *especially* skilled in manipulation. They have practiced this skill their whole lives and become very proficient.

Most people, including correctional professionals, are not naturally skilled at dealing with manipulation. This is often not a skill we've needed before coming to work in a jail or prison. But once there, learning to manage manipulation is an essential skill if you want to be happy in correctional practice. I call the art of dealing with manipulation *verbal jiujitsu*. To become a skilled practitioner of verbal jiujitsu, we must start with an analysis of what "manipulation" actually is.

Manipulation in a medical encounter occurs when a patient wants something he shouldn't have and won't take no for an answer. If the patient wants something he *should* have, no problem! Or if the patient is told no and accepts that answer, also no problem!

So manipulation involves these two essential elements:

1. The patient wants something she should not have. This something could be an extra mattress, a special diet, gabapentin, an MRI, a referral off site—anything.

2. The patient does not accept no for the answer.

What comes after not accepting no for an answer is *manipulation.* Manipulation is the attempt to coerce the practitioner into changing a *no* into a *yes.* Manipulation comes in many forms.

1. *Exaggeration*—"This is the worst pain in the world!" "I can't stand it any longer!" "I'm so much worse now than when I came to prison!" Exaggeration is an attempt to make this a special case, worthy of special consideration compared to other patients. "I know you usually say no, but no one else is hurting as much as I am!"

2. *Belittling*—"Only crappy doctors work in jails. No wonder you can't understand how to treat my pain syndrome. My outside doctor gave me what I need: oxycodone. Now *there* was a good and kind doctor! You should be ashamed." Belittling goes hand in hand with splitting.

3. *Splitting*—This consists of comparing you to someone else who would give the patient what he wants. The other person is commonly an outside practitioner. But splitting is especially effective when the other practitioner is someone within your own facility. "The other doctor who works at this prison gave an extra mattress to my cellie! And he's not in as much pain as I am!"

4. *Threatening*—This comes in various forms. First is the threat of physical violence. Patients can get quite skilled at communicating physical threats without saying a word. A particular hard look of tight jaw, narrowed eyes, tense muscles, and clenched fists, coming from a muscular guy with facial tattoos, can make anyone feel the hair stand up on the back of their neck, even if there is no way the patient could ever act on the threat. The second type of threat is various forms of complaints. Basically, the patient is saying, "If you don't give me what I want, I'll make your life miserable. I'll force you to comply with my will." Complaints may start with written grievances (that you must spend time and effort to answer) but then can quickly escalate to letters to the ACLU, formal complaints to your state board of medicine, pro se tort claims, and even malpractice lawsuits. Everyone who has worked in corrections for very long has heard the words, "You'll be hearing from my lawyer!"

5. *Fawning*—Fawning is, of course, the exact opposite of threatening and belittling. Fawning is more common with female patients, but males do it as well. "You're the best doctor I've ever met! I tell all the other girls in the pod how great you are!" Many patients are exceedingly good at fawning because, again, they have practiced their whole lives. A particularly insidious—and often effective—variation of fawning is flirting and sexual innuendo. "You always smell so good, Dr. Smith. What cologne do you use?" I remember one patient who told me, "Dr. Keller, you really know how to wear a suit. I worked at a clothing store, so I know."

6. *Filibustering*—Filibustering is being relentless in the demand that you change your mind. Filibustering is done in two distinct ways. Method No. 1 is this: "I won't leave your office until you give me what I want! I will argue with everything you say." An hour later the patient is still haranguing you, and your clinic schedule and nerves are both shot. Even more effective is the sequential strategy: "I will be in your clinic every week with the same complaint. Nothing you do (except for what I want) will ever work." After three, five, or 10 visits for the same complaint of "intolerable headaches," you might finally give in and write the prescription for gabapentin.

7. *The straw man victim*—The straw man tactic is where the manipulator charges you with acting against a protected class rather than based on your clinical findings. "You're only refusing me opioids because of my race/I am transgendered/I am Muslim," etc.

8. *The champion*—A *champion* is someone who pleads the patient's case from the outside. The champion can be an attorney or advocacy group but most commonly is a family member. Champions use all the manipulative techniques above, such as exaggeration, splitting, and incessant filibustering. Since champions are not incarcerated, they have access to many people whom patients themselves cannot easily reach, such as the sheriff, media, and even governor.

9. *Self-harm*—Self-harmers are patients who deliberately harm themselves to force you to do something they want. Examples include patients who cut themselves (*cutters*), *inserters* (patients who insert foreign bodies under the skin, into the penis, or anywhere they don't belong), and diabetics who try to induce severe hypoglycemic or hyperglycemic events in themselves. Self-harmers are often particularly hard to deal with.

HANDLING THE MANIPULATION OF CONFRONTATION

You are seeing a newly booked patient in your jail medical clinic. He says he's been in jails before, many times, and is always given a second mattress and an extra pillow because he had surgery on his back many years ago. You note the patient hasn't seen a doctor on the outside for many years, walks and moves normally, and has a normal neurological examination. You tell the patient medical does not give out passes for extra mattresses or pillows. The patient angrily erupts in a blaze of obscenities and threatens a lawsuit.

Manipulation happens when a patient wants something they should not have (like an extra mattress or pillow) and will not accept no for an answer. This patient is employing the strategy of threatening, one of several strategies patients may use to try to entice practitioners to change a no to a yes.

Verbal jiujitsu is the technique of deflecting and defusing manipulative confrontations. Notice I did not use the word *defeating*. That is because the first and most important rule of verbal jiujitsu is to remember this is not a war or contest! There should be no battle of wills between you and your patient. There is no winner or loser. Instead, you and your patient are having a conversation. The whole goal of verbal jiujitsu is to avoid any kind of verbal battle.

I know it's tempting to think of an unpleasant verbal exchange as a debate-style contest, with a winner and a loser at the end. In fact, sometimes patients try to provoke verbal fights as a strategy to get what they want. But even if you "win" a verbal battle, you actually lose because you've not accomplished your goal of getting your patient to understand and accept your treatment plan! Your patient is still not happy and will simply renew the verbal battle at another time in another way—and maybe more effectively next time.

The second rule of verbal jiujitsu is to maintain compassionate understanding of your patient. That person in front of you in your clinic is not an opponent or enemy to be defeated. He is your patient. Like everybody else patients are just trying to get by as well as they can in a very tough environment—they're incarcerated! It's just that many patients have poor interpersonal skills and resort to pathological social habits they've used their whole lives. This is what they know and what works for them. If a patient has successfully gotten his way over and over again by bullying and threatening others, that is how he will respond to you too.

You don't have control over this—but you do have control over your reaction. When patients confront you with threats, they will expect you to respond the same way most other people have responded—which is either to give in or fight back. These patients will be comfortable and practiced in handling either of these responses. You should do neither.

Take, for example, the case of this patient in your clinic who has angrily threatened to sue you, plus has lobbed in a few F-bombs for good measure. There he is, red-faced, fists clenched, and *loud*. Nurses, deputies, and other patients are watching. How are you going to handle this? How will you accomplish your goal of defusing the situation and facilitating reasonable communication with your patient?

Let's start with what you should not do.

The single worst thing you could do would be to respond to anger with anger: "You can't talk to me like that! Get the hell out! Who do you think you are?" First, the patient is accustomed to this type of response, is not surprised by it, and is far more effective at this type of confrontation than you are. The patient has now learned verbal confrontation is an effective way of getting under your skin. Plus, the fight is not over. The patient can (and will) renew the attack at another time. Also, you (hopefully) are not practiced and adept at angry shouting. You will have ruined your own mood for the rest of the day. How effective are you then going to be with the rest of your clinic schedule?

Another wrong response is to compromise: "There's no reason to be angry! Calm down, and we can work something out." Mistake! If you compromise, you have established the precedent that becoming angry is an effective strategy! The patient will threaten to do the same thing every time he wants something. And since every clinical encounter is discussed back in the dorms, other patients will also hear about this, and you will inevitably have to endure more confrontations.

Instead of these, defuse and deflect. One way would be to say, "I see you're angry, so we're done for now. Security will take you back to your dorm. We'll talk again later, after you've calmed down." It's important to say this without raising your voice and, if possible, betray no emotion with your face or body language. The lack of any reaction goes a long way to defusing such situations. No compromise, no bargaining, no reaction.

The next day—or even in an hour or two—you can call the patient back to medical and confidently expect a more productive conversation. It is important at this second interaction not to upbraid or belittle the patient. You should act as if the last incident is forgotten.

It takes training, practice, and time to master verbal defense skills. The best way to learn is through role-playing scenarios. The response to angry outbursts happens to be one of the easiest verbal jiujitsu skills to learn. The principles are: betray no reaction or emotion, end the session (if the patient will not calm down immediately), and make sure such patients know they are welcome back as soon as they calm down. Bring them back a short time later and act as if the incident is forgotten.

Is My Patient Faking?

I remember walking into one of my jails and seeing a patient on the floor of his cell, twitching and shaking. "Don't worry about him," said the sergeant on duty. "He's faking it."

Boy, that spun me up! Nothing will make me more anxious than hearing "he's faking" or its close cousin, "he's malingering." I hate and fear those words. Now, I know medical personnel, both in my jails and in the emergency departments where I used to work, get upset when they think they're being deceived or manipulated by a histrionic patient. But charging a patient with "faking it" is almost always a bad and dangerous idea.

There are three reasons for this. First, the charge of faking gets you and everyone else so emotionally charged up that no one is thinking clearly. Second, you might be wrong—and heaven help you if you are! Third, calling someone a faker is counterproductive to your real goal of getting the patient to stop doing whatever they are doing.

The first important consideration of calling someone a faker or a malingerer is that these words cause you and others to have a strong emotional reaction. When you say a patient is faking or malingering, whether you are correct or not, what that patient and others understand is that you're calling him a liar. This accusation elicits an immediate, powerful visceral response. You might argue, "I'm using the term *malingering* correctly according to its definition in the dictionary." Nobody will care. The patient and everyone else hear, "He's a *liar!*" Those are fighting words! When people hear those words, they stop thinking and go into fight-or-flight mode.

So, ask yourself this: *Is the medical information I'm conveying when I say a patient is faking so important that it outweighs the inevitable backlash of anger, frustration, and contempt?* Such emotions will ruin what otherwise might have been a fine day. But more important, they will get in the way of good medical practice. If you're feeling anger and contempt toward your patient, you're unlikely to provide stellar medical care for them—or for your next patient, for that matter. I don't know about you, but when I get angry and frustrated at work, my brooding sometimes makes me less attentive to my patients. And I might even go home and snap at my wife as well!

The second important item to think about before calling someone a faker is this: What if you're wrong? Most of the time you cannot know for sure whether a particular patient is deliberately faking or not. Consider, for example, a man in an airport who's having a panic attack about the prospect of getting onto an airplane. He is rocking back and forth, hyperventilating. His heart rate is over 150, and he is dripping sweat. He will not speak to those around him. These are dramatic symptoms, but I'd bet no one would say this man is faking it! His panic attack is real. With this in mind, are we 100% sure the patient in the jail cell who's twitching and incoherent is really faking it? If you get this wrong, you have a setup for disaster.

I have consulted on several medical liability cases in which patients were thought to be faking, were subsequently ignored, and had bad medical outcomes. If a patient is histrionic when he says, "My belly hurts," his dramatic presentation can be mislabeled as malingering, and his acute bowel obstruction will be missed. Similarly, "I can't breathe!" leads to, "He looks fine to me," which leads to, "He's faking." And pretty soon you're doing CPR. Anytime you hear the words "he's faking" or "she's malingering," you have entered an area of high medicolegal risk. Be wary!

But what about patients who really are faking their symptoms? There are admittedly a lot of these in jails and ERs. Let's assume our jail patient twitching on the floor really is faking his symptoms. Let's also assume he's doing this deliberately with the goal of getting out of jail, so he meets the definition of *malingering*. Now, correct me if I'm wrong here, but isn't our goal for him to stop faking? We want him to stop doing that twitch-and-moan thing and cooperate with us—in other words, behavioral modification. How likely is it that saying to him, "I know you're faking" will make him stop? To the contrary, malingerers who are accused of faking tend to redouble their efforts to convince you you're wrong and their symptoms are real! When a person has been publicly called a liar, he will want to regain his besmirched honor.

I have seen such patients try to force medical providers to believe them by being ever-present in clinics with the same complaint and by filing grievances and even lawsuits. Labeling a patient as a faker (even if you're right) has recast your relationship as adversarial. You are no longer on healthy terms as patient and caregiver. You are enemies now. How can anyone be on good terms with someone who has accused them of lying?

Let's return to our patient in the jail who is shaking and incoherent on the floor of his cell. There are three possibilities as to what is going on with him. He could indeed be faking. Alternatively, he could be having something akin to a panic attack, which, of course, is not the same thing as faking. Finally, he could be having a serious medical event. The only way to know is to do a complete medical evaluation and intervention. With enough patients like this, you're eventually going to see all three. With this patient no medical evaluation had been done. Once we did a physical exam and got vitals, we found he had a heart rate of 158, a blood pressure of 83/60, and a blood sugar of 875. Off to the ER he went with a diagnosis of diabetic ketoacidosis. This was a narrowly averted disaster.

How could this mistake have happened? Well, once the patient had been labeled a faker, rational thought ceased. Nobody considered the possibility they might be wrong! But another mistake was made as well: Doing nothing is the wrong approach, even if the patient is faking it.

Fortunately, there is one very good solution to this conundrum, and that is for us not to use the word *faker* even if we strongly suspect it. Don't even go there! There are other, better ways to approach histrionic patients with strange presentations. If we give up the judgmental attitude, we'll all feel better. More important, we'll also practice better medicine.

THE M-WORD—MALINGERING

I went to the always-excellent NCCHC (National Commission on Correctional Health Care) spring convention in Nashville a few years ago. One of the many outstanding presentations was done by frequent lecturer Deana Johnson. Deana talked about the risks of using the word *malingering*. Her basic message was to be very careful about saying an inmate is malingering—in fact, perhaps we should never use that word.

I was surprised by the degree of spirited disagreement from several members of the audience. They pointed out that *malingering* has a specific medical meaning, and sometimes—even often—it is an appropriate medical diagnosis. They pointed out that malingering is listed as an official diagnosis in *DSM-5* and that outside medical agencies like mental hospitals use the term. If we can't say an inmate who is clearly faking is *malingering*, what are we supposed to say?

It turns out there is indeed a correct and proper way to use the term *malingering* in correctional medical practice—but it is tricky and most often (in my experience) done incorrectly, with resultant bad consequences.

There are three important reasons for this. First, most people have an inaccurate idea of what *malingering* actually means in a medical sense and so use the term inaccurately. Second, the term also carries an emotional connotation that must be considered when it is used in a medical document. Finally, use of the term *malingering* has important consequences for patient relations, patient behavior, and time management.

The bottom line, in my opinion, is that *malingering* is a term that should very rarely be used in correctional medicine. There are better and more precise ways to convey medical information. But if you absolutely

The Best of Jail Medicine

want to use the term *malingering*, you need to know how to use the term correctly.

In my opinion, the most important consideration of the term *malingering* is not its actual definition. The most important part is its *emotional* meaning. This is a word that causes others to instantaneously have a strong emotional reaction. When you say a patient is *malingering*, whether you are using the term correctly or not, what that patient (and others) understand is that you are calling them a liar. This understanding is instantaneous and creates a powerful emotional response.

This emotional reaction places the word *malingering* in the company of other notorious words that generate emotional reactions that far overshadow their dictionary definitions. Examples are the N-word and the F-bomb. If you drop the F-bomb in your next professional case conference, you will not save yourself by arguing, "Well, I used the term correctly according to its definition in the dictionary."

Malingering is like this. *Malingering* is the M-word.

So ask yourself this: Is the information I'm conveying when I say a patient is malingering so important in a medical context that it outweighs the inevitable emotional backlash?

The Definition: Three Requirements

To answer that question, we need to look at the precise definition of the word *malingering*. Here is the Dictionary.com definition: *To pretend illness in order to shirk one's duty or avoid work.*

Here is a longer psychology definition: *The purposeful production of falsely or grossly exaggerated complaints with the goal of receiving a reward, such as money, insurance settlement, avoiding punishment, work, jury duty, the military, or some other kind of service.*

To satisfy this definition, you need to establish three things:

First, the patient must be pretending or feigning an illness.

Second, the patient must be doing this deliberately. It must be planned in advance.

Third, the patient must have the goal of obtaining something significant through the deception. Traditionally, malingering was done to shirk duty, such as military duty. In correctional medicine a comparable example would be to get out of jail or have charges dismissed.

Let's apply these to a couple of scenarios based on my own real-life experiences.

Feigning or Exaggerating?

Patient No. 1 has a history of back pain and back surgery. That led him into opioid addiction, which landed him in jail. He shuffled into my clinic bent over and limping because (he said) he was in so much pain that he could not function. The thing he needed was another back surgery, which could not be done while he was in jail. In the meantime, oxycodone was the one thing that worked for his pain, and he expected me to prescribe it.

When I declined this request, this patient became quite upset and stormed out of the clinic room threatening litigation. I couldn't help but notice as he left that he was not bent over and was no longer limping. He was striding along purposefully without any of the apparent disabilities he had before.

So here is the question: Was this patient malingering?

Well, to qualify as malingering, one must feign an illness. But based on my review of his MRI and surgical history, I have no doubt this patient truly did have low back pain. He wasn't feigning an illness he didn't have. Instead, he was exaggerating the disability this pain caused him. That is not technically malingering. Instead, this behavior is more properly described as *symptom magnification.* It would have served no purpose for me to say in the chart that this patient was malingering. Instead, I documented the discrepancy between the way the patient walked into the clinic and how he walked out and said it appeared there was no significant disability.

What good would it have done for me to use the M-word?

Calculated and Deliberate?

Here is a second example. A patient in my jail (we'll call him M.J.) said he must be released from jail because he had cancer of the blood diagnosed by a university cancer clinic in another state. He demanded to be released immediately so he could return to this out-of-state university to begin chemotherapy.

This is the sort of investigation the nurses in my jail love to do! In this case they discovered M.J. had indeed gone to this university cancer center claiming to have leukemia. However, a complete workup done there had been negative! The nurses also discovered this patient had been to several other cancer centers with the same claim and same result!

Would it be appropriate to say this patient was malingering?

The answer, again, is no. To qualify as malingering, M.J.'s deception had to be deliberate. In this case the patient truly believed he had cancer. His "cancer" was a persistent psychiatric delusion.

What Is the Goal?

I had a patient in my jails (Cory, let's call him) who faked seizures. These were not the psychogenic nonepileptic seizures I've written about before, but truly and deliberately faked (I know this because he eventually admitted it). Cory could do an excellent fake seizure, right down to biting his tongue and peeing his pants! Many patients with pseudoeseizures also have real seizures, but after extensive investigation, Cory was not one of them.

So—was Cory malingering?

Feigning a nonexistent medical illness—check. Doing so deliberately—check. But the goal being sought doesn't fit. Traditionally, malingering was done to avoid going into combat or going to work or to get a disability payment that was not deserved. But Cory had nothing that impressive in mind. Cory faked seizures because, well, he liked to fake seizures. He liked the attention and commotion and being in charge. Technically, this is not malingering. This is what is called *factitious disorder*. It would be incorrect to apply the M-word to Cory.

Here's another example. Throughout my career in both the ER and the jail, I have frequently encountered patients who have some variation of this common complaint: "I have chronic pain, and the pain medication I'm being prescribed isn't working. I need something stronger, like _____." (Fill in the blank here: oxycodone, tramadol, gabapentin, Lyrica, etc.)

In this case, even if I can show they are grossly exaggerating the degree of their pain, the goal being sought does not qualify. If what the patient wants is stronger pain medication than you are offering, that does not qualify as *malingering*. This behavior is so common that to call it the M-word would negate the meaning of the word. The goal has to be greater than med-seeking, at least in my mind.

In the end it can be truly hard to know for sure that a patient is malingering. You have to be able to say it's not symptom magnification— the patient really has no symptoms at all. You have to be able to say the patient is perpetrating this falsehood knowingly and deliberately. And you have to know what it is the patient wants—something more than better painkillers. When you use the M-word, you are rendering a final judgment about all these things.

What if You're Wrong?

This is the single most important item to think about before you use the M-word: What if you're wrong? One of my ER partners had a young man present with sudden atraumatic loss of feeling and function from his waist down. He seemed weirdly unconcerned about this sudden catastrophic development. His interaction with his parents suggested attention seeking. Most patients with such a story end up being diagnosed with a conversion reaction or factitious disorder or some other psychiatric cause. My partner sent him home, telling the parents "He's faking." Only… he wasn't. This patient had a rare congenital AV malformation and was indeed a new quadriplegic. You can guess the result of this fiasco: lawsuit. Recriminations. Disciplinary actions. It got ugly.

What Is the Goal?

Correct me if I'm wrong, but for all these patients I've presented here, the true ultimate goal is for them to *stop*! Stop exaggerating your symptoms! Stop believing you have cancer when you don't! Stop faking seizures! Stop bugging me for stronger pain meds you shouldn't have!

How likely is an accusation of malingering to affect this goal? Here is what I believe: If you accuse a patient of malingering, that patient is unlikely to stop. In fact, I think they will be more likely to do the exact

The Best of Jail Medicine

opposite and accelerate their complaints to convince you they're telling the truth. They will want to regain their besmirched honor! In fact, many of them will try to force you to believe them, via grievances, lawsuits, and being ever-present in your clinic.

Simply by using the M-word, you have redefined your relationship with these patients as adversarial. From a time-management standpoint, you will now spend a lot of time arguing, answering grievances, and attending case management meetings.

I venture to say none of this is really what you want! Getting these patients to stop their egregious behavior requires behavioral modification techniques, which is a totally different kind of verbal jiujitsu. The M-word does not appear in these techniques.

In the end, in my opinion, medical practitioners in corrections should rarely, if ever, use the word *malingering* in their documentation. Most of the time the cases we're talking about do not meet the strict definition of malingering. Also, we do not want to be enemies with our patients. Enemies may retaliate by using grievances and lawsuits.

Use of the M-word will tend to make inappropriate behaviors worse when we want them to stop. Using the M-word will almost invariably be a time drain because you will have to repeatedly justify its use, over and over and over again.

It's just not worth it—most of the time.

CHEMICAL SEDATION VS. PHYSICAL RESTRAINT

Here's the clinical scenario: You have an inmate in your facility who is running his head into wall, bull-like, at full speed. He backs up and does this repeatedly. He may be suicidal. He may be high on meth. He may just be a jerk throwing a tantrum. But he will not stop just because you ask him to.

What would you do in this situation? It seems to me there are only three options for how to deal with this inmate.

1. Do nothing! Let him hurt himself if he wants.
2. Physically restrain him in a restraint chair or on a board.
3. Administer medications to achieve chemical sedation.

These three responses clearly are different in their risk of a bad outcome. And there are two possible bad outcomes to consider. The first is the medical risk. Which approach is most likely to result in a serious injury to the patient? The second is the legal risk. Which approach is least likely to result in a successful lawsuit?

I hope no one reading this would opt to do nothing. You simply cannot continue to let this inmate run his head against the wall. The risk of a bad outcome, both medical and legal, is just too high. On the medical side, I personally am aware of three cases where inmates running their heads into the walls of their cells fractured their necks. One was left a quadriplegic. The risk of legal action is also high. In fact, this could be deliberate indifference: You knew running his head into the wall could potentially result in serious injury and yet did nothing to stop him. I will leave the deliberate indifference question to the lawyers, but even without this, the threat of a nasty lawsuit following such an injury is almost inevitable.

So the prudent action, both medically and legally, is to restrain this patient in some way. But which method of restraint is safer for the patient? Which method is safer legally?

In my strongly held opinion, restraint by chemical sedation is safer than prolonged physical restraint for those who are a threat to injuring themselves or others. I have several reasons for believing this.

- Chemical sedation is the community standard of care in the other two areas of medicine that also routinely restrain patients who are threats to themselves or others, emergency medicine and inpatient psychiatric medicine.
- Prolonged physical restraint, for example in a restraint chair or board, carries significant risks of injury, including death. Chemical sedation is much safer.
- As long as the chemical sedation is done properly, there is less risk of successful legal action with chemical sedation than with prolonged physical restraint.

The Community Standard of Care

I practiced in a busy emergency department for many years before I came to correctional medicine. There, chemical sedation was routinely practiced. Every emergency department does chemical sedation routinely. It is not controversial in ERs at all. I was taught how to do chemical sedation in my ER residency. It is an emergency medicine core competency. Chemical sedation is discussed in every major emergency medicine textbook. As a matter of fact, physical restraint is viewed in emergency medicine as a tool to facilitate chemical sedation rather than a viable option on its own.

It is similar in inpatient psychiatric hospitals. I have asked several psychiatrists whether they leave dangerous inmates in a psych hospital physically restrained for long periods of time. The typical response is to laugh and say, "No. They get sedated."

I'm not sure why chemical sedation has such a bad reputation in some quarters of the correctional medicine world, because it is the standard of care for patients who are an acute danger to themselves or others elsewhere in medicine. Why is this so? It is because *chemical sedation is safer than prolonged physical restraint.*

Unfortunately, I cannot point to any published studies that show chemical sedation is safer than prolonged physical restraint. That is because there are none. However, I personally know of at least five cases of death from physical restraint. The mechanism of death in these cases has ranged from suffocation to acute pulmonary embolism to "excited delirium." The point is that prolonged physical restraint carries substantial risks that range from minor (contusions, abrasions, broken bones) to serious (death, loss of limbs from too-tight restraints).

On the other hand, I am not aware of any deaths from chemical sedation, whether in an emergency department setting or in corrections. I actually have never heard of any serious complications from chemical sedation.

Legal Risk

I have spoken to several different risk management experts on the subject, in both emergency and correctional medicine, and they have unanimously agreed that chemical sedation of dangerous patients carries less legal risk than prolonged physical restraint.

Here is one example. I contacted Rick Bukata and Greg Henry, who together publish *Risk Management Monthly*, a publication on how to reduce medicolegal risk in emergency departments. I asked them about the legal risk of administering chemical sedation to a dangerous patient against his will. This was their response:

"This situation is not likely to be problematic if the patient is being sedated because he or she poses a danger to self or others and if the reason for sedation is meticulously documented. A physician might be at greater medicolegal risk if he or she fails to sedate a problematic patient who is placing the staff in jeopardy."

After talking to several risk management experts in correctional medicine about this subject, I am unaware of any successful lawsuits arising from chemical sedation of an incarcerated inmate who was an acute danger to himself or others. If you are aware of such a lawsuit, I want to know about it!

I believe the legal risk of restraining an inmate depends on two factors. The first is harm. If a patient has been harmed by the restraints, he is more likely to sue and more likely to be successful. So the method of restraint least likely to injure the patient is the safest legally. Chemical sedation is safer than prolonged physical restraint and so is safer legally as well.

The second factor is that the sedation is done on the right patient (one who is an acute danger to himself or others) and that this is documented properly.

In fact, chemical sedation is like administering any medication: You must have the right patient, give the right medications in the right dosages, do the right monitoring and follow-up care, and document in the right way. If you do all of that, your legal risk will be low.

OPINIONS

The Meaning of Medically Necessary

Let's say one of my jail patients has a moderate-size inguinal hernia. I want to schedule surgery to have the hernia fixed, but to do so, I have to get authorization. This is not unusual. Just like the outside, before I can do medical procedures or order nonformulary drugs, I must get the approval of the entity that will pay the bill. By contract my jails house people from a variety of jurisdictions, such as the federal marshals, ICE, the state department of corrections, and other counties. This process of "utilization management" is very similar to getting preauthorization from an insurance company or Medicaid in the free world, probably because corrections simply copied the outside preauthorization process.

Having done this process hundreds of times over the years, both in the free world and in correctional medicine, I am struck by a phrase that keeps coming up: *medically necessary*. When authorization for a procedure is denied, the reason often given is that it is "not medically necessary." I then have to argue that what I am requesting is, indeed, medically necessary. The problem is that there are many possible definitions of *medically necessary*, and I believe many disagreements arise because two parties understand medical necessity differently.

Medically necessary might mean *necessary to sustain life*. In other words, without this procedure or treatment, the patient will or is likely to die. For example, insulin is medically necessary for type 1 diabetics. Without insulin they will die. Dialysis is medically necessary for patients with no renal function; otherwise they will die. Chemotherapy is medically necessary for the survival of cancer patients. Surgery is medically necessary for perforated bowels. However, this definition leaves out many therapies where the benefit is harder to quantitate.

Is insulin medically necessary for a type 2 diabetic? Is Flomax medically necessary for a man with urinary difficulty? Is surgical repair medically necessary for a torn rotator cuff? By this definition probably not. This is the definition likely to be used when the reviewer wants to deny a claim. *Necessary to sustain life* is great when you don't want to pay for a procedure or a medication. But using this definition can reach absurdity. I once saw a man who had been incarcerated in prison for many years prior to being transferred to my jail. When I first examined him, I found an inguinal hernia so large he had intestines in his volleyball-size scrotum. I asked, "Why haven't you ever had this hernia fixed?" I asked. "They told me it wasn't medically necessary."

This is the definition utilization management people have in mind when they deny treatment for hepatitis C in patients with no evidence (yet) of liver disease.

This definition clearly is not the right one for correctional medicine.

Medically necessary might also mean *commonly done in the community.*

This "community standard" is probably the most common definition for *medically necessary* I hear when people discuss medical treatment for jail patients. It sounds good: If a patient can get a procedure or medicine in the community, it should also be available in prison. That seems to make sense. However, there are problems with this.

The first is that what is commonly done in the community depends on the patient's insurance status. Take a surgical repair of a torn rotator cuff, for example. A well-insured patient will have that surgery done. A patient with no insurance will not. Rotator cuff repair is a surgery hospitals and surgeons will not do without payment. They justify this by reverting to "it's not necessary to sustain life."

A second problem with the "community standard" is that many medical treatments commonly done in the community have no solid foundation in science. Many expensive medications commonly prescribed are no better than less-expensive generics (like just about everything in the typical medication cabinet). In 2020 the *Journal of the American Medical Association* published a paper worth reading titled "De-adopting Low-Value Care: Evidence, Eminence, and Economics" that advocated eliminating commonly done but low-value medical care.[1] This is also the goal of the Choosing Wisely Campaign, in which representatives of various medical specialties were asked for lists of medical tests and procedures that were commonly done in the community but should not be.[2] These are fascinating to read through. A good place to start is the Choosing Wisely recommendations of the American Academy of Family Physicians.[3]

Community standard is so easy to meet that it is the definition people reach for when they want some medical procedure approved. For this very reason the community standard should not be the go-to definition of *medically necessary*. It is too lax—it allows too much low-value and even harmful medical care.

Medically necessary might mean *accepted medical practice*.

Accepted medical practice means the medical procedure or treatment is recommended by an up-to-date medical textbook (like UpToDate or Essential Evidence Plus) or a guideline published by a legitimate medical group (such as the U.S. Preventative Services Task Force or American Academy of Family Physicians). This (in my opinion) should be the standard definition of *medically necessary*. Ideally, if I want authorization for something, I should be prepared to back my request up with a credible source. If a procedure is denied, I expect the denier to be able to cite a medical source as the reason.

Of course the reality is messier than this ideal of looking everything up! One problem is that many published guidelines are not evidence-based, unduly influenced by Big Pharma, or otherwise simply crappy.[4] A third problem is that many topics in medicine are controversial. Some good physicians will do one thing, and other good physicians will do another.

Finally, the people who do utilization management reviews (usually RNs) are sometimes not familiar with the medical literature. That is why many UM decisions are outsourced to proprietary "evidence-based" algorithms such as McKesson's InterQual or the MCG (Milliman Care Guidelines).

For me, knowing the various definitions of *medically necessary* helps me in my quest to get surgery approved for my patient's hernia. This surgery may not be necessary to sustain life, but it is the community standard of care (no community surgeon will ever say, "Nope, I don't want to fix that!"), and surgery is the recommended treatment by medical textbooks and guidelines.

References

1. Powers BW, Jain SH, Shrank WH. De-adopting Low-Value Care: Evidence, Eminence, and Economics. *JAMA*. 2020; 324(16): 1603–4. doi:10.1001/jama.2020.17534
2. Choosing Wisely. Accessed May 21, 2022. www.choosingwisely.org
3. Choosing Wisely. Clinician lists: American Academy of Family Physicians. Accessed May 21, 2022. www.choosingwisely.org/clinician-lists/#parentSociety=American_Academy_of_Family_Physicians
4. Costa Molina CdR, leite-Santos NC, Gabriel FC, et al.; for the Chronic Diseases and Informed Decisions (CHRONIDE) Group. Factors Associated With High-Quality Guidelines for the Pharmacologic Management of Chronic Diseases in Primary Care: A Systematic Review. *JAMA Intern Med.* 2019; 179(4): 553–60. doi:10.1001/jamainternmed.2018.7529

COVID-19 Fatigue and Leadership

When COVID-19 burst onto the scene in early 2020, the administrators and medical teams in my jails initiated several commonsense practices to reduce the possibility of COVID infiltrating the jails. These included screening and quarantining new patients before allowing them into the dorms, screening jail employees daily, doing lots of COVID tests, and, perhaps most important, having deputies wear masks at work. That helped us avoid major COVID problems at my jails.

However, I quickly noticed growing evidence of "COVID fatigue" in my community. When I'd go out in public, I was one of the very few still wearing a mask. And this unfortunately spilled over to the correctional facilities. I did a clinic at one of my smaller jails a few months into the year and was surprised and dismayed to see the deputies were no longer wearing masks. In the meantime community COVID cases were climbing, so the risk of transmitting COVID to the jail was actually greater than it was, say, a month earlier.

What remained constant throughout the pandemic was that the greatest risk to jail patients was not new incarcerated people with COVID but deputies or other jail employees catching COVID in the community and bringing it to the jail before knowing they had it. One of such jail personnel is me! I also had a responsibility not to be a potential COVID vector. That meant wearing a mask at the jail, but it also meant I had a responsibility to practice COVID safety in the community.

I thought of it this way: Of every 1,000 people I met in my community (most of whom I didn't already know), at least one was statistically likely to have COVID. The best way to prevent transmission from that person to me was for that person to be wearing a mask. This was unlikely where I live, though.

The next best way to prevent transmission from that person to me was for *me* to wear a mask, practice social distancing, and clean my hands often. These actions would lessen the likelihood that I'd catch COVID and transmit it myself into the jail. My job is to keep the people in my jails healthy. In the time of COVID, my actions when I'm not at work impact my primary goal of keeping my jail patients healthy. If I didn't practice COVID safety in the community, I'd be abrogating my duty just as assuredly as if I failed to provide necessary medical care.

I also have a powerful leadership role whether I want it or not. If a jail deputy were to see me at the store without a mask, that would reinforce their perception that "this COVID thing isn't that big a deal." Same thing with many of my friends who get their medical information from political sources. They know I'm a physician, so when they'd see me wear a mask, it would reinforce that wearing a mask in public is an important medical practice.

So, keep yourself safe! Keep your patients safe! Exercise a positive leadership role in your community through leading by example! Do all of these by embracing safe practices around COVID-19 and other transmissible threats at work and in the community.

A CONCRETE CELL FOR THE MENTALLY ILL

Consider the case of a 60-year-old patient I'll call "Library Man." While at the public library, Library Man took off most of his clothes and was talking loudly to no one in particular. The police were called, of course. He was charged with disturbing the peace and brought to my jail.

Jails basically have three types of housing areas. First are dormitory-style rooms with 60–100 residents. Library Man could not be housed there—the young, aggressive inmates might prey on him. Second are smaller cells that hold 2–4 people. The problem with these cells is that even if the jail could guarantee gentle cellmates, it would be hard to monitor Library Man in such cells. Such cells tend to be in out-of-the-way places and have small windows on the doors. The only place Library Man could be reasonably housed in most jails is "special housing," which refers in this case to a single-man isolation cell with lots of plexiglass to allow easy observation. Such rooms are designed to contain nothing someone could use to harm themselves, so they are made entirely of concrete and steel—even the bed. This is where Library Man ended up—basically in a large concrete box.

Unfortunately, this was not a good place for Library Man to be. You may have guessed Library Man was a homeless schizophrenic who had gone off his meds. He was harmless—certainly not a danger to himself or others. In his psychotic state he did not understand why he was arrested and jailed. Library Man would have benefited from familiar surroundings and normal social interaction with people. He got neither of these in the alien and sterile environment of his concrete isolation cell.

I should make it clear here that I am not criticizing the jail. The jail medical and mental health personnel do what they can to help people like

The Best of Jail Medicine

Library Man. They'll get him back on his medications. If necessary, they'll coordinate commitment proceedings. The jail social worker will work with outside psychosocial rehab services to help transition him back into the community. Library Man was eventually released after three weeks in jail.

My point is that Library Man should never have gone to jail in the first place. He was a harmless (though disruptive) mentally ill man. The jail was never designed to house the seriously mentally ill. The reason Library Man came to jail is that in my state, as in many others, funding for mental health services was severely cut several years ago. As a direct result Library Man and many others lost access to mental health services. Consequently, my jails saw a marked increase in the number of mentally ill patients like Library Man being brought there.

The police officer who responded to the call from the library recognized Library Man was mentally ill. But the local for-profit psychiatric facility would not take Library Man. The state psychiatric hospital was full and would only take him after a long commitment process anyway. The local crisis center wasn't staffed to handle someone as sick as Library Man. The only option left to the police was to take Library Man to jail. And the jail had nowhere to put him except the concrete cell of special housing.

Sadly, Library Man is not an isolated case. Another recent patient housed in special housing was a developmentally delayed woman who had hit one of her caregivers at her shelter home. She was an adult in body but probably only 8 years old or so on a functional level. She also did not understand why she was in a cold concrete room. "I want my dad!" she wailed. The jail staff tried to calm her with coloring books and Pikachu stickers during her several-day stay.

Jails and prisons have become the resource of last resort for the mentally ill, just like emergency rooms have for people who cannot afford healthcare. It should not be this way. A concrete room at the jail is not the right place for people such as Library Man or Developmentally Delayed Girl to be. It is not in their best interest. It is not a wise use of the jail facility or staff.

And it is expensive! Multiply the cost of housing Library Man times the hundreds of thousands like him incarcerated in our jails and prisons currently. That money would easily pay for effective community programs to keep the mentally ill out of incarceration.

What's the solution to this problem? I confess I don't have the answers. The first step, though, is to recognize that a problem exists. What happens inside the walls of a jail is often invisible. It needs to be made public. Is this really what we want?

How Lawsuits Drive Correctional Medicine

Imagine, if you will, a nurse assigned to take care of 50 patients on a medical floor—by herself. Clearly this is an impossible task. There are just too many patients for one nurse to adequately monitor. But this nurse gamely does her best.

Now let's say there's a bad outcome and an investigation. Even if the understaffing problem is recognized, it would be easy—and tempting—to scapegoat the nurse, especially if there was no intention of fixing the staffing problem ("We can't afford to hire more nurses!"). Instead the scapegoated nurse would be replaced by a new nurse, who, once again, would be expected to care for 50 patients.

Such were my thoughts when I read a 2019 *Chicago Tribune* article about the problems with the medical care for patients in the Illinois prison system.[1] The article said there had been so many problems with medical care in the Illinois prison system that a class action lawsuit successfully forced the state to make sweeping changes. What is not mentioned in the article is that similar lawsuits have happened before in other states and will happen again.

It starts here: The main factor that results in poor medical care in prison systems in the United States is that prison systems tend to be severely underfunded. Because they are underfunded, prison medical systems are almost universally understaffed, especially with nurses but also with medical practitioners. Medical personnel do their best, but if you are working in a prison and trying to shoulder the workload of 2–3 FTEs, well, it might not always turn out well.

So how did prisons end up in this situation?

Funding and staffing for medical care have not kept pace with the huge increases in the sheer number of incarcerated patients that began in the 1970s. This is also true of other parts of the prison systems, such as housing. Many state prison systems are severely overcrowded.

The prison patient population is getting older and sicker. Older and sicker patients will, of course, need more medical care than a young and healthy cohort. Funding for medical care in prisons has not kept pace with the aging of incarcerated patients.

Nursing wages have risen steeply in the last several years. Prisons are competing with hospitals, outside clinics, and everyone else for nurses. In general prisons do not pay enough to be truly competitive. Prisons are hard paces to work and so should pay commensurately higher wages than, say, hospitals. But this is not the case in most prison systems. As a result it is not unusual for a typical state prison system to have, say, a third of its nursing positions vacant.

Medical care in the United States is getting more and more expensive, and prison budgets have not kept pace. Examples are plentiful, but here is a good one: Treatment for hepatitis C is now highly effective but also very expensive. The prevalence of hepatitis C in prison populations averages around 18%. To treat every one of them with a treatment that costs many, many thousands of dollars apiece—well, you do the math for your state. It is a lot.

So why has funding for prison medical systems not kept pace with the needs of incarcerated patients?

Because such funding has to be approved by each state's legislature. And this is often a hard sell. Legislators may ask, "Why are we spending millions more on prison healthcare when many of my unincarcerated constituents can't get health insurance?" This is a reasonable question. Plus, free constituents vote! The incarcerated generally do not. A legislator who introduces a bill to, say, fund millions for hepatitis C treatment for prison patients may not be a legislator for long! Prison medical care is a political "poison pill."

This is why increases for prison healthcare funding often are driven by lawsuits. Since the Supreme Court has ruled that incarcerated people have a constitutional right to necessary medical care (Estelle v. Gamble, 1976), a lawsuit that shows that jail or prison patients are not receiving adequate medical care will usually win. And this opens the door for legislators to write the check for increased prison medical funding without having to pay a political price. "I had to vote for this even though I didn't want to," they can say to constituents. This has happened many times in other states before Illinois and will continue to happen in the future.

In nutshell, then, this is our dysfunctional relationship with prison medical care in the United States: As the incarcerated population rises and patients get older, funding for their medical care becomes inadequate. This results (among other things) in understaffed medical services. Legislatures won't increase medical funding because that would be politically untenable. With time, underfunding and understaffing lead to bad medical outcomes. Advocacy attorneys then file class action lawsuits on behalf of incarcerated patients alleging inadequate medical care—and win. This forces legislatures to increase funding for medical care, which they can now do without paying a political price. And then the cycle repeats.

This cycle is being played out over time in most U.S. states, probably including yours. So don't be surprised by the next inevitable news article about a successful lawsuit that forces a state to increase funding for prison medical care. That is how the system works.

Reference

1. Lourgos AL. Accused of preventable inmate deaths, state agrees to sweeping health care reforms, oversight at all prisons. *Chicago Tribune.* Published January 4, 2019. www.chicagotribune.com/news/breaking/ct-met-illinois-prison-health-lawsuit-20190103-story.html

Can the Raiders Be Saved Using the Principles of Medical Research?

One of my good friends is a die-hard Las Vegas (previously Oakland) Raiders fan. In 2018 the franchise fell on some hard times. The Raiders went from being one of the best teams in the league in 2016 to one of the worst in 2018, with a dismal 4-12 record. As a result my friend had to suffer taunts from fans of better teams (like me!). He became despondent.

But it doesn't have to be this way! That year's Raiders could have quickly and easily turned things around by using the tried-and-true techniques of medical research. If a pharmaceutical company did 16 clinical trials of their new potential blockbuster Drug X, they would never let a 4-12 outcome get them down. When published I guarantee those trial results would look a lot better than 4-12. We can use the same technique to improve the Raiders' record. Keep these methods in mind when you review medical research from the correctional or any other setting.

Change the Primary End Point

Before a medical study begins, the researchers must identify exactly what they are studying. This is called the *primary end point.* For example, the researchers studying Drug X could initially decide their primary end point is whether Drug X reduces mortality over five years. What happens, though, if the study shows Drug X does not, in fact, reduce mortality? Well, in that case researchers will often scrutinize their data to find out if Drug X showed some other benefit they were not initially looking for.

Let's say that patients taking Drug X had fewer DVTs. This finding may have resulted purely by chance, but what the heck! They could publish a paper that says Drug X reduces DVTs without mentioning this was not the original primary end point of their study. It turns out this practice is common in published research papers and is called *outcome switching.*

According to a recent survey, outcome switching occurred in over 50% of the papers studied.[1]

In a football game the primary outcome is, of course, the final score. The Raiders lost 12 games in the 2018 season using that primary outcome. But if we look closely at each of these 12 games, we might be able to find another potential outcome we could switch to. Take, for example, when the Raiders played the Indianapolis Colts on October 28, 2018. The Raiders lost that game 42-28. But if we were to switch the outcome to the score at the end of three quarters, the Raiders won 28-21! We'll publish that as a victory without saying we changed the primary outcome. Similarly, in their second game of the season, the Raiders lost to the Denver Broncos 28-20. But if we change the outcome to the score at *halftime*, we can publish this as a win, 12-0! We can do the same thing for their first game against the Los Angeles Rams.

After changing these primary outcomes, the Raiders' record has improved to 7-9. We're on our way!

Use Composite Outcomes

If a pharmaceutical researcher isn't sure if Drug X will get positive results in any particular primary end point—like death, for example— they may instead add multiple other end points, hoping to get a hit on at least one. The additional end points could include heart attacks, strokes, or anything else they can think of, like DVTs or even inpatient hospital days. If any one of the many composite outcomes comes up positive, then the whole study can be published as positive. Of course, a DVT is much less important than, say, death, but since both are listed as equals in the composite end point, you would have to really read the fine print to find out if the "hit" was death or DVTs.

Composite end points turn out to be an immensely useful tool in reevaluating the Raiders' 2018 season. My composite end points for the Raiders' games are these: final score, total yards, first downs, and time of possession. I applied these composite end points to each of the Raiders' remaining losses. Take, for example, the third game of the season, against the Miami Dolphins. The Raiders lost that game 28-20, but they had more total yards, more first downs, and a longer time of possession. Clearly, we can publish this as a victory for the Raiders using our composite end points. Applying our composite end points, we can similarly change five other losses to victories.

The Raiders' record now is 13-3.

Simply Don't Publish the Negative Results

This has long been the easiest and best way to bury a negative trial: Simply don't publish it! Negative studies in the medical literature have long been much less likely to be published than positive studies. This publication bias has been such a big problem in pharmaceutical research that in 2004 many medical journals started requiring studies to be preregistered in a clinical trial database. This ensured negative studies could be tracked even if they were not published. So, is this requirement working? Not so much. A report 10 years later found publication bias still alive and well.[2]

Publication bias can certainly help the Raiders. Their revised 2018 season still includes three losses. And all three were embarrassments, where the Raiders got their butts kicked. Take the October 14th game against the Seattle Seahawks, for example. Not only was the final score a lopsided 27-3, but the Seahawks had far more total yardage, more first downs, more everything. Let's forget that debacle by simply not publishing it! Let's not publish the other two losses, either.

The Raiders' record now is 13-0. However, we're still not done. The Raiders played 16 games, not 13. We still must find three other positive outcomes…

Publish a Positive Study More Than Once

If a medical researcher has a positive study, it can be tempting to publish the results in more than one medical journal. That way the researcher gets two citations in their résumé for the price of one! There are two ways to do this. The first is to submit the same data to multiple journals without telling them you have done so. Duplicate publication like this is a form of fraud but more common than you think.

Another way to get a study published multiple times is to publish only part of its data and then later publish the rest in a second article. For example, in our study of Drug X, we could publish the data showing the effect of the drug on mortality first and then later publish the data showing the effect on DVTs. If the study is large enough and the researchers slice the data thin enough, they can get many publications out of a single trial.

Let's apply this principle to the Raiders. Their most impressive victory of the 2018 season was when they upset a very good Pittsburgh Steelers team on December 9th. We certainly want to publish that twice! Let's also duplicate-publish the Raiders' victories over the Denver Broncos and Cleveland Browns.

Well, we're finished. The Raiders' final record after applying the principles of medical research is an undefeated 16-0! My friend can break out the champagne and let the celebration begin! And to all of you other long-suffering Raiders fans out there—you're welcome.

References

1. Jones CW, Misemer BS, Platts-Mills TF, et al. Primary outcome switching among drug trials with and without principal investigator financial ties to industry: a cross-sectional study. *BMJ Open.* 2018; 8: e019831. doi: 10.1136/bmjopen-2017-019831

2. Walsh N. RA: Publication Bias Alive and Well. Medpage Today. Published August 27, 2014. www.medpagetoday.com/rheumatology/arthritis/47386

About the Author

Jeffrey E. Keller, MD, is a board-certified emergency physician who was asked by his local county commissioners in 1997 to provide medical care to the local jail. With the addition of more jails and juvenile facilities, the company Badger Medical was born and Dr. Keller learned correctional medicine was his true calling. Dr. Keller went on to supervise medical care in several state prison systems. He began writing the very successful blog Jail Medicine in 2012. He was awarded the Armond Start Award of Excellence for work in correctional medicine by the American College of Correctional Physicians in 2020. Dr. Keller is now retired from correctional medicine but continues to cheerlead from the sidelines. He lives in Idaho Falls, Idaho with his wife, Angela, reading lots of books and doing a deep dive into gardening.

Made in the USA
Las Vegas, NV
02 December 2022

60913546R00105